NEW MEDICAL FRONTIERS

Patient's Practical Guide

>>><<<

Manage
Cancer Treatment
SIDE EFFECTS
Naturally

BASED ON MORE THAN 200 DIFFERENT
NATURAL REMEDIES AND MODALITIES
SCIENTIFICALLY VALIDATED BY MORE THAN
400 U.S. & INTERNATIONAL MEDICAL SCHOOLS
& RESEARCH INSTITUTIONS

Dr. Mark Fritz, NMD, PhD

>>><<<

Disclaimer

The information given in this guide is for informational purposes only and is not intended to replace the advice and treatment by a healthcare provider. This is especially true for recommended dosages (that are just a reference points). Work with your physician to determine the safest and most effective dosage for you.

All contents of this book are commentary or opinion and are protected under Free speech laws in all civilized countries. The information is provided for educational and entertainment purposes only and is not intended to diagnose, treat, cure, or prevent any condition or disease. Dr. Mark Fritz assumes no responsibility for the use or misuse of this material. No warranty of any kind, whether expressed or implied, is given in relation to this information or any of the external services referred to. This is a comprehensive limitation of liability that applies to all damages of any kind, including (without limitation) compensatory, direct, indirect or consequential damages.

Instead of an own

FOREWORD

"The doctor of the future will give no medicine, but will interest his patients in the care of the human body, in diet and in the cause and prevention of disease."

Thomas Alva Edison
America's most prolific inventor in history

>>><<<

Doing justice accordingly, this publication is primarily for patients to be best informed and who are interested in self-management ('self-efficacy') of their health.

Following the Harvard University *Health Letter*
(Volume 32/Number 6/April 2007/p. 7):

"Patient, manage thyself"

Contents

Introduction

When you are diagnosed with cancer, as a first step, your oncologist may consider following basic modalities to get you on remission: surgery to remove a tumor, as well as chemotherapy and/or radiation to destroy as many cancer cells as possible. Since, on one side, the human body is a strictly natural-biological phenomenon, and on the other, the synthetic oncologic procedure is highly toxic, this incompatibility leads to many debilitating side effects as a kind of 'defense' of your body.

If these side effects, again, are treated with synthetic-chemical drugs and modalities, the vicious cycle closes – with risk of premature death. Only recently, the Queensland University of Technology in Australia, has published the results of a landmark study, according to which driving 'under influence' of prescription drugs is no less dangerous as driving under the influence of illegal drugs, and culpable in a crash.

To circumvent this fate and still relieve and overcome these side effects, this book features **more than 200 different natural remedies and modalities – complementary** to your oncologic treatment. These are not only historically evidence-based, but have been **scientifically validated** (science-based) by **more than 400 medical schools and research institutions in the U.S. and international** (see list provided in *References*).

Please note that generally there are no guarantees, no warrantees, and no *one-size-fits-all in* medicine. Still, this guide may well be your best chance to relieve and overcome side effects of conventional cancer treatment, naturally.

It is vital for any patient to have a basic up-to-date knowledge with respect to his/her health problem at stake, being the master of his/her most valuable asset: *health*. Doing justice accordingly, is the mission of this **patient's** guide.

>>><<<

This is the first volume of a series of Patient's Guides
"New Medical Frontiers"
in the field of Natural Medicine

SIDE EFFECTS

OF CONVENTIONAL
CANCER TREATMENT

Appreciating the reality that our body is a highly complex ecosystem strictly dependent on natural laws, any medical treatment which is not in line with these natural laws, will harm your body in one or another way ('side effects').

This is especially true for radiation, as well as chemotherapy, prescribed to about 80% of cancer patients in the U.S., with highly cytotoxic drugs – regardless if administered orally or intravenously (IV) to slow tumor growth and destroy as many fast proliferating tumor cells as possible.

Since these cytotoxic cannot differ among fast proliferating cells, they destroy also other fast proliferating – healthy – cells – such as hair cells and cells of the stomach lining. That's why side effects like, inter alia, hair loss, nausea, vomiting, digestive disorders – and above all: suppression of your body's inherent natural *immunity* - are a logical consequence.

Just as the *Immune Recovery Clinic* in Atlanta, GA, put it:
"Cancer cannot exist in a fully intact immune system."

Unfortunately, you cannot relieve and overcome these side effects with other synthetic/man-made chemicals but only with natural modalities and substances.

Natural remedies – as validated by folk medicine and nowadays by scientific studies – are in line with your biological status with following advantages:

- No or very few side effects
- High safety and efficacy
- Much lower cost than patented drugs

Special reference is given to our globe's biggest natural pharmacy: the Amazon *Rainforest,* where the author has been trained.

In addition this guide is focusing on herbs well known, and appreciated, in *Traditional Chinese Medicine* (TCM), and those known in Indian natural Ayurvedic medicine.

The positive effects of these 'exotic' herbs are evidence-based, which is most valuable. They have been used successfully by indigenous inhabitants for centuries, if not millennia, as advised by their natural 'doctors' (shamans, etc.).

According to the World Health Organization, even today 80% of the world population relies on herbs for their health. In many cases as *centenarians* (i.e. life expectancies of more than 100 years – like the peasants high up in the South American Andes).

In the very best interest of straightforwardness and direct access to the recommended remedies, their historic-medical background is not explained in detail in each case in this book.

The recommended dosages are just reference points, only. How much to take depends on your individual situation. Work with your physician to determine the safest and most effective dosage for you.

There may well be drug interactions, as some natural herbs may have the same efficacy as synthetic/chemical prescription drugs and may – in that case – potentiate the efficacy. If you are on any prescription drugs, please contact your healthcare provider before using herbs.

As you will see in the following, there is usually more than one remedy listed for a specific side effect. Which one is right in your specific case? This is an issue of trying out, as 7 billion inhabitants of this globe have 7 billion different metabolisms. There is no 'one-size-fits-all' in medicine. Rather, you have to find the best way for your personal problem in the context of your individual actual circumstances.

In cases where specific remedies are recommended for more than one side effect, do not multiply the respective dosage: one remedy, one dosage.

Also, please note: If you want to make use of herbs, always consider using the whole herb and not an extract, if possible. Preferably drink it as a tea (infusion) or decoction (simmering), because the hot water extracts the active components from the herb best.

All remedies recommended in this guide are basically available in the U.S., many of those online.

ANEMIA

Our body's blood circulation – in fact the transport system for nutrients and oxygen to support all cells in our body – besides platelets and plasma, consists of 2 types of blood cells: red (99%) and white (1%).

While the red blood cells carry oxygen through the body, giving the blood its red color, and remove carbon dioxide from the body, the 1% white blood cells, center part of our immune system, are protecting our health by fighting bacteria and viruses responsible for infections, thus protecting us from illness and disease.

Conventional cancer treatment such as chemotherapy and radiation is decreasing red blood cells for oxygen support, thus compromising your body's self-healing power which alone can overcome cancer at all. We call that *Anemia* known in medical history since 4000 years..

What are the potential causes and side effects becoming anemic with conventional cancer treatment?
Inter alia,

- Surgery
- Chronic inflammation & anti-inflammatory drugs
- Hormonal imbalances
- Nutrient deficiencies in terms of
  - minerals (especially iron, also in combination with manganese) and
  - vitamins (especially B-9/folic acid, B-12, and C)
- Drug use (with special reference to chemotherapy and radiation), that's why conventional cancer treatment is especially responsible for anemia.

Fatigue is the no. 1 symptom of Anemia, besides many others, like cognitive impairment due to iron deficiency, according to research at *Pennsylvania State University*. And scientifically validated by, inter alia, the *Nemours Foundation* in Jacksonville, Florida.

To counterbalance anemia, you may well refrain from chemical anemia drugs with lots of side effects, including the risk of thrombosis specifically for cancer patients. As scientifically validated at the *New York Presbyterian Hospital* and *Columbia University Medical Center*.
Also, a dietary supplement 'multi' is not the best choice.

Instead, as a first step get a blood count to identify your deficiencies with respect to anemia, in terms of vitamins (especially *B-12, B-9/folic acid* & *C*) and minerals (most important *iron,* in combination also with *manganese)* and the trace mineral *selenium* to re-balance your blood count again.

Then, go natural especially with fruits and vegetables supporting this natural process. Inter alia,

- *Apples*
- *Plums*
- *Apricots,*
- *Purple Grapes*
- *Spinach*
- *Beets*
- *Squash*
- *Whole Grains*
- *Legumes*
- *Beef liver*
- *Chicken liver*
- *Fish*
- *Poultry*

In case of iron specifically, these foods are an excellent source:

- Liver
- Lean beef
- Seafood (oysters, shrimp, clams, tuna)
- Fruits (figs, dried apricots, prunes, raisins)
- Vegetables (spinach, greens, beans, avocados, broccoli, peas, lentils)

ANXIETY

According to research at, inter alia, the *University of Western Ontario,* Canada, anxiety affects every 6th person worldwide, many of those life-long. Still, it is one of the most misinterpreted *mental health conditions* today, according to the *Imperial College* in London.

With a wide spectrum of symptoms like dizziness, nervousness, chest pain, heart palpitations, insomnia, dry mouth.

Panic attacks are an intensified situation in many cases, or at least felt as such according to the *University of Granada* in Spain, in general last some 30 minutes, and in rare cases even hours, according to the *American Psychological Association.*

Anxiety is also strongly linked with *depression* and *stress* - making them, together with *mood disorders*, the predominant causes of *chronic illness* (with special reference to cancer), according to the *World Health Organization (WHO).*

A similar link has been revealed between *immunity* and *anxiety,* based on research at *Columbia University* and *Rockefeller University*, both located in New York City.

In terms of cancer, anxiety has a specifically high impact when it comes to false results of screenings – which happens frequently – according to comprehensive research at *Skane University Hospital* in Malmo, Sweden.

Therefore, it is not only essential but vital, to get a *second opinion* if the first screening turns out positive, since screenings are all but perfect.

According to research at *Rockefeller University* and *Columbia University* in the U.S., anxiety has a major impact also on the immune system.

Even worse, according to scientific findings at the *University of Warwick* in Coventry, UK, anti-anxiety drugs incorporate a risk of premature death.

While psychiatric therapies have not solved this severe health problem yet, same is with side-effect-intensive medications, nature has developed remedies over thousands of years, especially in Indian *Ayurvedic medicine* and *Traditional Chinese Medicine (TCM).*

Probably the most important herb, according to the *University of Michigan* and the Indian *CSM Medical University*, is

- **Ashwagandha** (Botanical name: Withania somnifera)

known in *Ayurvedic* medicine for more than 3000 years not only as *anxiolytic* (anti-anxiety) but also, inter alia, as immune-boosting, anti-stress, anti-inflammatory and anti-tumor. With special reference to chemotherapy and radiation – according to research at *McMaster University* in Canada.

Recommended daily **dosage** 2 times 500 mg.

- **Chamomile** (Botanical name: Matricaria chamomilla)

is an excellent remedy for relieving anxiety.

Recommended daily **dosage** up to 350 mg.

Similar the results for

- **Passion Flower** (Botanical name: Passiflora incarnate)

both according to research at, inter alia, the *University of Maryland*.

Recommended daily **dosage** up to 4 times 250 mg each.

Also,

- **Roseroot/Golden Root** (Botanical name: Rhodiola rosea)

an arctic root from originally Siberia, has great reputation to ward off anxiety, depression, and stress, according to research at the *University of Pennsylvania* and *Columbia University*.

Recommended daily **dosage** up to 300 mg.

Excellent reputation to relieve anxiety, depression and cognitive decline has the bark of

- **Magnolia** (Botanical name: Magnolia stellata)

according to the *Institute for Traditional Medicine* in Portland, Oregon.

Recommended daily **dosage** 30 mg.

Also, according to research at the *American Herbalist Guild*, a daily cup of tea from

- **Peppermint** (Botanical name: Mentha piperita)
  &
- **Elderflower** (Botanical name: Sambucus nigra L.)

 can reduce anxiety because of its antimicrobial power.

Essential

- **Peppermint Oil**

helps also for anxiety and fatigue, according to the *Jesuit University* in West Virginia.

Another powerful remedy for relieving anxiety (and stress) is the amino acid

- **L-Theanine**

as scientifically validated, inter alia, at *Cleveland Clinic* in Cleveland, OH, and the *University of Shizuoka* in Japan.

Recommended daily **dosage** up to 250 mg.

Please note that L-theanine is part of **green tea**.

Similar the results for the herb (from a pepper plant)

- **Kava** (Botanical name: Piper methysticum)

as scientifically validated at, inter alia, *South Dakota State University*.

Recommended daily **dosage** of 3 times daily 100 mg or up to 400 mg twice daily.

However, since Kava has been questioned by FDA in late 2001/early 2002, based on potential liver problems in Europe with reference to Kava (however, without banning it in the U.S.), you may check with your healthcare provider, if this herb is good for you, which dosage exactly, and how long you should take it.

Also, the hormone

- **DHEA** (Dehydroepiandrosterone)

plays a positive role in the process of relieving anxiety naturally.

According to research at *Yale University*, the *Veterans Administration National Center for Post Traumatic Stress Disorder* and the *Veterans Affairs New England Healthcare System* in West Haven, CT.

Recommended daily **dosage** 100 mg.

Another powerful remedy is

- **Vitamin B-complex**

With special reference to Vitamin B-1 which can relieve anxiety and support mental clarity according to, inter alia, Dr. Janet Travell, a professor from *George Washington University Medical School*, and former physician for Presidents John F. Kennedy and Lyndon Baines Johnson at the White House.

Vitamin B-3 (Niacin) offering similar results as so called *Nature's Valium*, and highly deficient in our population as well.

Same as Vitamin B-6 (Pyridoxine), Vitamin B-5 (Pantothenic Acid), and Vitamin B-12.

Recommended daily **dosage** for Vitamin B-complex see label.

Equally important is

- **Magnesium**

so called 'anti-stress mineral' of which most Americans are highly deficient in their food, with approximately only half of the recommended **dosage** of up to 500 mg. Scientifically validated, inter alia, at the international *Kumamoto University* in Japan.

- **Physical Exercise**

in terms of physical aerobic activity is helpful, as your brain produces *endorphins* which make you 'happy' – the natural way. (Refrain from legal and illegal drugs promising the same result!)

Because aerobic exercise at least 20 minutes 4 times weekly supports energy, blood circulation, and synthesis of hormones such as cortisol important for a sense of well-being. As scientifically validated, inter alia, at the *University of Montana* in Missoula.

Finally, you may follow a century old natural therapy nowadays scientifically validated, inter alia, at *Walter Reed National Military Medical Center* – turn to

● ***Music***

to relieve anxiety at home or wherever you are. What kind of music? Just what you like most! When and how long? You decide.

This self-administered therapy is specifically helpful to relieve anxiety and pain before, at, or after surgery, according to research at *Brunel University* in the UK.

>>><<<

See also chapters
DEPRESSION, MOOD SWINGS, STRESS

BLOOD CLOTS

Blood clots, i.e. blood cell (platelet) stickiness, along with poor blood circulation due to high blood viscosity in arteries and veins, thus cutting off blood with vital nutrients and oxygen from heart, brain, and lungs, are responsible for the biggest health problem in our civilization.

There are some 5 million cases in the U.S. per year, along with 800,000 hospitalizations. Leading to more than 1 million deaths annually, not to talk about amputations of arms and legs.

Heart-related deaths due to blood clots alone cause more than 700,000 deaths per year, followed by some 200,000 deaths as a consequence of blood clots in legs, and some 170,000 because of blood clots in the brain. The latter is also responsible for 80% of strokes.

When it comes to cancer, this situation is even more dramatic, as research at, inter alia, *Leiden University* Medical Center in Leiden, the Netherlands, and *King's College* in London, UK, proved according to which cancer patients have an up to seven-fold increased risk for blood clots in legs or lungs. (Venous thrombosis.) For cancer patients with distant metastases, the risk is increasing.

The underlying cause of cancer-induced blood clots is cytotoxic drugs such as *cyclophosphamide* used in *chem*otherapy.

According to research at, and validation by *King's College* in London, UK, and the *Swedish Research Council* in Stockholm, the risk of blood clotting is even higher with prostate cancer patients.

However, unlike widespread myth, chemical drugs cannot solve this problem, because of the side effects involved, like bleedings in the gastrointestinal tract or brain, macular degeneration, or bone fractures, caused by certain blood-thinning drugs. As scientifically validated by, inter alia, Canadian *McMaster University* and *St. Joseph's Hospital,* both in Hamilton, Ontario. That's why the FDA has launched a serious warning.

Fortunately yet, more than 3000 years ago, in Japan

- **_Nattokinase_**

an enzyme fermented from soybean derivate *natto* has been found to be an excellent blood thinner (with no debilitating side effects), which can dissolve blood clots even in hours. Nowadays scientifically validated by, inter alia, the *Center for Natural Medicine* in Portland, OR, and the *University of California* in Davis.

Recommended **_dosage_** 100 mg 1-2 times daily.

In our hemisphere, the herb

- **_Ginger_** (Botanical name: Zingiber officinale)

derived from the rhizome and consumed as a tea has an excellent anti-platelet reputation. Based on research at the *University of Michigan, University of Rochester* in Rochester, NY, and the *Royal Hospital for Women* in Sydney, Australia. Scientifically validated by the *Memorial Sloan Kettering Center* in New York.

Recommended daily **_dosage:_** 2-3 cups of tea or up to 1 g powdered.

Another helpful remedy is

- **_Lycopene_**

a carotenoid pigment giving vegetables and fruits their red color. Like tomatoes and watermelons. According to *Rowett Research Institute in* Aberdeen, Scotland.

As an appropriate **_dosage,_** 2 to 4 tomatoes should be eaten, which is an equivalent of up to 40 mg Lycopene daily.

Same effect, according to research at *Tufts University,* may be reached with eating onions containing a sulfur-type molecule.

Also, a daily cup of

- **_Cocoa_** (botanical name: teobroma cacao)

can well keep blood clots and their dramatic/fatal consequences away by inhibiting the platelet process, as scientifically validated, inter alia, at *Southampton General Hospital* in Southampton, UK.

Similar results have been achieved at Beltsville Human Nutrition Research Center's Phytonutrients Laboratory of *Auburn University* in Auburn, Alabama, with Chinese

- **Wolfberry** (Botanical name: Lucium barbarum)

and

- **Sweet Peppers**

Equally beneficial for blood flow to the brain is

- **Beetroot Juice**

according to scientific findings at *Wake Forest University* in North Carolina.

Similar the effect of

- **Virgin Olive Oil**

which reduces platelet aggregation, according to a study conducted at the *University of Malaga* in Spain.

As another Mediterranean health food,

- **Garlic**

is beneficial to ward off blood clots, according to scientific validation at Albert Einstein College of Medicine at *Yeshiva University* in New York City, NY.

Going back to 2-times Nobel Prize laureate Linus Pauling, former professor at *Oregon State University*,

- **Vitamin C**

is basically helpful to fight cancer, but it may also prevent thrombosis with a **dosage** of 500 mg 4 times daily.

Based on research at *Harvard University*, funded by the U.S. Institutes of Health, also

- ***Vitamin E***

can prevent venous thromboembolism (VTE).

Recommended daily ***dosage*** up to 1000 IU.

Eating

- ***Oats***

is also beneficial for preventing blood clots, according to *Tufts University* in Boston, funded by the U.S. Department of Agriculture.

And for those who like it more 'technical', at the 18th National Symposium on Endovascular Therapy in Miami Beach, Florida, in January 2006, the *Baptist Cardiac and Vascular Institute,* Miami, has introduced a new

- ***Ultrasound***

device small enough to slip through blood vessels with a hair-thin wire, dissolving blood clots in the legs and pelvis.

CACHEXIA

The harsh chemical and radiological tools of conventional oncologic treatments are basically the contrary of what the ecosystem of your biologically well defined body and mind need. That's why these modalities lead to *remission* – not a cure – at best.

There are dramatic side effects, including *cachexia* – a more or less complete waste of your body – with weight loss and muscular dystrophy (sarcopenia), because of malnourishment caused by an accelerated protein breakdown. Comprehensively researched at, inter alia, Ohio *State University.*

In fact, cachexia is not an illness or disease but a complex metabolic syndrome in strict sense, of which 80% of cancer cases are affected, and 40% die of.

To relieve this fate, there are quite a few natural remedies to apply. Such as

- ***Omega-3 (Fish Oil)***

according to research at, inter alia, *RWTH Aachen University* in Germany.

Recommended daily ***dosage*** up to 1000 mg daily.

As well as the amino acids

- ***L-Glutathione***

and

- ***L-Arginine***

based on research at the *University of Bridgeport*, CT.

Recommended dosage up to 100 mg daily for L-Glutathione and 3 times daily 1000 mg for L-Arginine.

>>><<<

See also chapters
IMMUNITY WEAKNESS, MALNUTRITION, INFECTION

CHEMO BRAIN

Unfortunately, *chemotherapy* (a term coined in the early 1900s by its inventor, the German chemist Paul Ehrlich) not only attacks cancer cells, but any fast proliferating cells like hair cells (causing hair loss) and of the stomach lining (causing nausea and vomiting). They also attack the central nervous system and *brain* cells. The latter leading to forgetfulness and loss of concentration in a seemingly fuzzy head.

More than half of patients on chemotherapy have only 10% of the cognitive performance – at best – according to School of Psychological Science at the *University of Manchester*, UK.

This is a realistic impact, which many doctors deny, disregarding the fact that – yes – these highly toxic drugs can cross the blood-brain barrier. Scientifically validated by *University of British Columbia* in Canada, as well as the *West Virginia University* School of Medicine and by the *Radiological Society of North America* (RSNA).

Since FDA has not approved any drug to treat this phenomenon of chemo brain, some doctors prescribe, inter alia, 'off label' drugs they usually prescribe for ADHD (Attention Deficit & Hyperactivity Disorder) – with no positive result.

However, there are some encouraging natural alternatives such as

- *Ginkgo* (Botanical name: Ginkgo biloba)

which supports a healthy brain and memory,

and

- *Ginseng* (Botanical name: Panax ginseng)

as recommended by *Mayo Clinic*.

(Recommended **dosage** up to 100 mg daily for Ginkgo and up to 500 mg daily for Ginseng.)

Along with a recommended daily **dosage** of up to 1000 IU of

- *Vitamin E*

Another herb to relieve 'chemo brain', based on research at the *University of Wollongong* in Australia, and historically known in Indian Ayurveda natural medicine and *Traditional Chinese Medicine* (TCM) is

- *Bacopa* (Botanical name: Bacopa monnieri)

Recommended daily *dosage* up to 500 mg 1-3 times daily.

Also encouraging is the amino acid

- *Acetyl-L-Carnitine*

according to research at the *Institut de Cancerologie de l'Ouest* in Nantes, France, and the *Memorial Sloan Kettering Cancer Center* in the U.S.

Recommended daily *dosage* 500 mg 1-2 times.

Another prospective amino acid to be used for chemo brain is

- *L-Theanine*

a substance in green tea – according to U.S. *Memorial Sloan Kettering Cancer Center* and the *University of Shizuoka* in Japan.

Recommended *dosage* 200 mg twice daily.

- *Coenzyme Q10 (CoQ10)*

a vitamin-like antioxidant in some foods and in supplement form may also relieve chemo brain according to research at David Geffen School of Medicine at the *University of California* in Los Angeles.

Recommended *dosage* 200 mg 1-2 times daily.

- *Phosphatidylserine* (PS)

supports a healthy mind.

Recommended daily *dosage* 100 mg.

PS is found in many foods with different content (from potato – 1 mg per g) up to soy lecithin (with 5900 mg per 100 g).

CONSTIPATION

Constipation, is derived from the Latin word *constipare* coined 1400 A.D., for irregularity, meaning 'press, crowd together'.

According to *Mayo Clinic,* every third adult citizen in the U.S. is chronically constipated, characterized by only 2 or less bowl movements per week, and hard stools. And some 2.5 million doctor visits per year. With commercial laxatives worsening the situation.

This way, the U.S. today is the most constipated country in the Western world, with a dramatic effect on highest ranking chronic ailments such as heart failure, cancer, obesity, diabetes, intestinal disorders.

In terms of cancer, constipation is usually the result of chemotherapy and radiation – besides of the possibility that a tumor may affect the digestive system. Especially conventional medications for pain and chemotherapy may cause constipation.

To relieve this phenomenon which is not only a matter of convenience and life quality, but also of a strong immunity and hormone balancing, lifestyle changes may be the first choice – according to research at, inter alia, *Johns Hopkins University,* the *University of North Carolina* in Chapel Hill, and *Mayo Clinic* in Minnesota.

Start lifestyle changes with increasing (aerobic)

- ***Physical Exercise***

such as walking, tennis, swimming, jogging, volleyball) to stimulate the colon (scientifically validated also at *Johns Hopkins University),*

along with eating 15-20 g of (soluble and insoluble)

- ***Fiber***

a day (corresponding to 2 servings of high-fiber bran cereal), and drinking more

- ***Fluids***

like 8 glasses of water (8 oz. each), and also fruit juices.

Scientifically validated at *Johns Hopkins* University in Baltimore, MD, and the *University of North Carolina* in Chapel Hill, N.C.

The deficiency of both (lack of fiber and fluids) is the main reason for constipation, according to the *American Society of Colon and Rectal Surgeons.*

While cheese, eggs, meats and other high fat foods (like fast food) are low in fiber, whole grains, fruits (especially dried figs), vegetables (especially broccoli), legumes (especially cooked black beans and lentils) as well as nuts (especially almonds) are an excellent source for a diet rich in fiber. According to the *University of Toronto,* validated by the U.S. Department of Agriculture.

Also

- **Psyllium Husk** (Botanical name: Plantago Psyllium)

may help according to research at *McGill University* in Montreal, Canada, and the *University of Toronto.*

Recommended daily **dosage** up to 500 mg.

According to the *U.S. Department of Agriculture,* best sources of fiber are

- **Fruits**

    such as

  ➢ Figs, dried
  ➢ Raspberries, raw
  ➢ Prunes
  ➢ Pears, with skin

- **Vegetables**

    such as

  ➢ Broccoli, cooked
  ➢ Brussel Sprouts, cooked
  ➢ Artichokes, cooked
  ➢ Sweet Potatoes, baked in skin

- *Grains*

  such as

  - Barley
  - Brown Rice
  - Couscous
  all cooked

- *Nuts*

  such as

  - Almonds
  - Pecans
  - Peanuts

  and

- *Beans*

  such as (all cooked)

  - Black Beans
  - Pinto Beans
  - Kidney Beans
  - Navy Beans

Also, the freshwater algae

- *Chlorella* (Botanical name: Chlorella vulgaris)

as a marine plant relieves constipation, according to research at *Mimasaka Women's College* in Okayama, Japan.

Recommended daily *dosage* of 1000 mg.

DEHYDRATION

Water – you can't live without. Since it makes up more than half of your blood and body weight, and it is undeniable vital for *all* functions and biochemical reactions your body needs to perform, day and night.

Despite of that, one third of Americans are chronically dehydrated. Caused by the fact that, because of sedentary lifestyle, our body does not automatically 'require' enough water as it did, e.g., when working physically in the field before the Industrial Revolution took place.

Although there are signs we mostly ignore (or misinterpret) such as, e.g., slight headache, *constipation* due to hardened stools, dry eyes, fatigue, dry mouth, dizziness.

Not to overlooking the fact that, yes, you are losing water during sleep.

There are considerable health risks, including **cancer** of the breast, colon, and the urinary tract), according to research at, inter alia, the *University of Washington* in Seattle, WA. Also, dehydration is concentrating chemical medications in the body, leading to, inter alia, poor kidney function, and toxicity and, yes, even dementia – one of our society's increasing health problems.

This situation getting even worse with diuretics and other medications which upset the water balance in the body.

Not to forget about dehydration as a consequence of chemotherapy and radiation, with special reference also to medically caused vomiting.

To avoid this 'ride on the hamster wheel', you should get at least 48 ounces of liquids (8 glasses 6 oz. each) according to, inter alia, *Tufts University* research - preferably spring water, potentially including fruit and vegetable juices with high content of water such as, inter alia, watermelon, celery, tomatoes, radishes, cucumbers, and cauliflower.

DEPRESSION

Depression is the leading cause of disability with some 350 million cases worldwide.

According to research at the *University of Western Ontario,* Canada, depression is strongly linked to *anxiety* and *stress.* Together with *mood disorders*, these are the predominant causes of *chronic illness,* according to the *World Health Organization (WHO).*

Similar the results of a study elaborated at *Duke University* in Durham, N.C., proving a potential link between depression and *diabetes.*

Unlike most diagnoses coming up with a checklist of different symptoms, depression is in fact a complex and complicated health problem which needs to be seen as such – validated by researchers at the *Catholic University* in Leuven, Belgium. Most healthcare providers handle different symptoms individually, without appreciating any interrelations – especially psychological ones like depression.

Even worse, depression is strongly related to cancer in around half of cases (with lung cancer patients on top of the list), because of the life-threatening psychological implications of this diagnosis. Still, almost 3 quarters of depressed cancer patients do not receive depression treatment. As scientifically validated by the *National Institute for Mental Health* (NIMH) – the largest scientific institution of this kind worldwide – in Rockville, MD.

This is especially problematic, as depression in many cases hinders the affected patients to get cancer treatment at all. And there is an increased risk of death when both conditions correlate and depression left untreated – as scientifically validated by the *Geisel School of Medicine* in Hanover, NH, supported by research at the *University of British Columbia* in Canada. (A vicious cycle!)

As pointed out already, our body (and mind) is a complex/systemic/inter-related phenomenon. Accordingly, different ailments can be strongly related to each other. As an example you may take *anxiety, depression, eating disorders, memory loss, mood swings, fatigue, sleep disorders.* Still, we do not recommend 'one-size-fits-all' in terms of remedies; rather go individually by the respective ailment.

Since you may not only suffer from depression but also other related ailments, this does not mean to add the respective dosages of the very same remedy.

As explained already by other examples in this book, man is a systemically interconnected phenomenon ('ecosystem') which is not easily understood at first glance. This implies, however, that links between certain ailments are not necessarily understandable at first glance.

One of those biological 'secrets' not easily understood is the scientifically validated fact that *diabetes* raises depression. According to research at *Beth Israel Deaconess Medical Center* and *Brigham & Women's Hospital,* both in Boston. Added by research at the *University of Washington* School of Medicine in Seattle, according to which diabetes and depression together are a risk factor for Alzheimer's and dementia.

This example of biologic interrelations demonstrates that, even if you believe this or that side effect is not related to conventional cancer treatment, and it is not covered in this book, don't overlook this side effect.

Unfortunately, it is a tremendous myth to believe that commercial anti-depressant drugs – 3rd most prescribed drugs after painkillers and cholesterol statins – can handle this problem.

Rather, there are more than 70 (!) dangerous – and in many cases long-term – adverse effects known for anti-depressants. Many of those chemical drugs even worsen the situation. One of these adverse effects is thickening of arteries with the risk of heart attacks and stroke, according to, inter alia, *Emory University School of Medicine*, and the *University of Queensland* in Australia.

Another risk is bleedings in the brain, according to research at *Western University of London*, Ontario in Canada. Also, anti-depressant drugs incorporate the risk of birth defects, according to the *National Center on Birth Defects and Developmental Disabilities* at the U.S. governmental *Centers for Disease Control and Prevention (CDC)*.

Not enough, according to research at the *University of Liverpool* in the UK, there is no scientific proof for 85% of depression treatments recommended by National Health Service in the UK to work at all.

Therefore, the best way to get off this 'hamster wheel' is with natural modalities.

As an example, since most cases of depression found in cancer patients are stress-related,

- **Physical Exercise**

is strongly recommended. This way your brain produces *endorphins* which make you 'happy' – the natural way. (Refrain from legal and illegal drugs promising the same result!) And it helps you to feel better 'from the inside out'.

According to research at the *Karolinska Institute* in Sweden, and the *Center for Mind-Body Medicine* in Washington, D.C. Scientifically validated at the *University of Texas*, recommending 45-60 minutes a day, 3 to 5 times a week.

However, according to, inter alia, the *Boston University* School of Medicine, just *walking* may not suffice, as this kind of movement does not produce enough brain chemicals to improve your mood and does not let you be less anxious.

Same research base – *Boston University* – also recommends to practice

- **Yoga**

for mood enhancing by stimulating parts of the brain and increasing the brain chemical gamma-aminobutyric acid (GABA) as a neurotransmitter which, to be sure, you can also add separately as a dietary supplement.

However, although GABA is to be found in some commercial anti-depressants, you may refrain from that version which, to be sure, is not natural but synthesized, and mixed with other synthetic chemicals (a vicious cycle).

A deficiency of

- **Vitamin B-9 (Folic Acid) & Vitamin B-12**

which can lead to depression, according to research at the *Department of Psychiatry of the Hospital District of Southern Savo* in Finland. Therefore, your levels of folic acid and vitamin B-12 should be checked as well by a comprehensive blood count as well.

One of the multiple factors which may support the development of depression also in cancer patients is a deficiency of

- ***Vitamin D***

according to research at, inter alia, *Oregon State University*, the *University of Texas Southwestern Medical Center* in Dallas. Validated by U.S. *Mayo Clinic, Oregon State University*, and the *University College London* in the UK

Therefore have your blood count checked with special reference to Vitamin D deficiency.

Vitamin D enhances survival chances in many cases, cancer included – according to research at the *University of Edinburgh* in the UK. To overcome a deficiency of this essential nutrient which also supports immune function and is existential especially when cancer has been diagnosed, moderate exposure to sunlight is the best source of vitamin D, as our skin (regardless which part of our body) produces vitamin D at sun exposure. For second choice, take nutrition like milk and oily fish.

In terms of herbs,

- ***Ashwagandha*** (Botanical name: Withania somnifera)

the ancient herb used since 3000 years in India's natural medicine *Ayurveda*, is at least as effective as any chemical drug – just without side effects. Validated, inter alia, by research at the *Toyama Medical and Pharmaceutical University* in Japan.

Recommended daily ***dosage*** up to 500 mg.

As another recommended herb

- ***Roseroot/Golden Root*** (Botanical name: Rhodiola rosea)

an arctic root from originally Siberia has great reputation to ward off depression, anxiety, and stress, according to research at the *University of Pennsylvania* and *Columbia University.*

Recommended daily ***dosage*** up to 300 mg.

Excellent reputation to relieve depression, anxiety, and cognitive decline has the bark of

● ***Magnolia*** (Botanical name: Magnolia stellata)

This is known for some 2000 years and has been validated by, inter alia, the *Institute for Traditional Medicine* in Portland, Oregon.

Recommended ***dosage*** 30 mg.

● ***Black Cohosh*** (Botanical name: Actaea racemosa)

is also a valuable herb to relieve depression. Based on research at, inter alia, *The University of Montana* in Missoula.

Recommended ***dosage*** up to 40 mg twice daily.

You may miss in this context so far

● ***St. John's Wort*** (Botanical name: Hypericum perforatum)

This is an example why a *personalized* therapy is absolutely essential – if not vital.

Especially as it is the leading herb for depression in the U.S. The reason for our cautiousness despite of its reputation is research at *Wake Forest Baptist Medical Center*, according to which possible drug interactions may occur.

E.g., it could cause heart disease because of impaired efficacy of hypertension (high blood pressure) medications, or lead to an unwanted pregnancy due to failure of contraception. In this case, however, the contraindicative problem lies with the chemical drug, not the natural nutrient.

Recommended ***dosage*** up to 300 mg daily.

Another potent option for depression relief is the nutritional supplement

● ***S-Adenosylmethionine (SAMe)***

according to research based on a clinical trial at the *University of Queensland* in Australia.

Recommended daily ***dosage*** up to 1,600 mg.

Also, as a natural – and essential – nutrient to relieve depression

- **Omega-3**

is recommended in form of polyunsaturated fatty acids to be consumed preferably as fish oil. It has a positive effect on the brain function. According to joint Anglo-Iranian research at *Teheran University of Medical Sciences.*

Not only this, regular

- **Fish**

consumption in your diet can keep depression at bay, according to research at *The Medical College of Qingdao University* in Qingdao, China.

As an excellent example how closely related body and mind are, consider

- **Probiotics**

to fight depression (and stress disorders) with – and that's probiotics all about – live bacteria in your digestive system. According to research at, inter alia, the *University College* in Cork, Ireland. Probiotics are fermented food such as yogurt.

Also, research at *Plant & Food Research*, Auckland, New Zealand, in cooperation with *Northumbria University* in the UK, shows that

- **Blackcurrants**

(at least those grown in New Zealand) increase attention capacity and mood, and are therefore recommended for depression.

The probably most innovative scientific finding on how to prevent and relieve depression comes from the *University of Las Palmas de Gran Canaria* in Spain, according to which

- **Mediterranean Diet**

with lots of fruits and vegetables is not only healthy physically but may also have a positive effect mentally – depression included.

Finally, you may follow a century old natural therapy nowadays scientifically validated, inter alia, at *Walter Reed National Military Medical Center* – by turning to

- ***Music***

to relieve depression at home or wherever you are. What kind of music? Just what you like most! When and how long? You decide.

This self-administered therapy is specifically helpful to relieve depression as well as anxiety and pain before, at, or after surgery, scientifically validated also at *Brunel University* in the UK.

DIGESTIVE DISORDERS

According to the *American College of Gastroenterology* in Las Vegas, more than 60 million Americans have a rebellious digestion once in a while – with, inter alia, heartburn, dyspepsia, gastro esophageal reflux disease (GERD), irritable bowel syndrome (IBS), or diarrhea. They spend more than $1 billion/year for over-the-counter (OTC) medication. When becoming chronic, it can develop cancer.

To have or not to have a good digestive system is a matter of health of your *intestinal flora* (mostly made up of some 100 trillion good bacteria).

This implies that good and bad bacteria in the gut need to be balanced to avoid development of typical chronic conditions nowadays such as metabolic syndrome, obesity, chronic fatigue syndrome, diabetes, rheumatoid arthritis, allergies – and *cancer*.

In addition gut bacteria can reduce gastrointestinal effects of chemotherapy according to research at, inter alia, the *University of North Carolina* in Chapel Hill. This is especially true for *Icaritin*, one of most prescribed chemo drugs which, however, causes *diarrhea* in 90% of cases.

Not only this, a balanced system of gut bacteria can delay age-related diseases in general, according to a recent study elaborated at the *University of California* in Los Angeles (UCLA), funded by the *National Institutes of Health' National Institute on Aging*.

Therefore, it is very essential – not to say *vital* – to incorporate **probiotics** with friendly bacteria *Lactobacillus acidophilus* and *Bifidobacterium longum* in your daily regimen – at least by supplementing, better with Yoghurt.

Unfortunately yet, different lifestyle issues and medical problems may deteriorate your intestinal flora and digestive system, respectively, according to, inter alia, *Johns Hopkins University* and *Feinberg School of Medicine of Northwestern University* in Evanston, Illinois.

While more than half of American adults are diagnosed with digestive disorders, they rely on over-the-counter (OTC) antacids.

However, unlike what you may have been advised otherwise, digestive drugs cause digestive distress and an increase of stomach acid. When this acid gets into the esophagus – we call that *heartburn*. If it gets chronic, it can lead to *Barrett's esophagus* and – yes – even to esophageal cancer.

Also these drugs may cause side effects such as diarrhea and weakened bones. A vicious cycle!

This could be balanced out naturally with a combination of

- **Zinc**

and the amino acid

- **L-Carnosine**

according to research at the *University of Hong Kong,* scientifically validated at *Akita University* in Japan and the *Medical College of Georgia* in Atlanta, GA.

Recommended daily **dosage** 75 mg twice daily.

When talking about nutrients for better digestion, we should also consider one specific herb, sometimes called one of the best-kept health secrets of the world, and this is

- **Curcumin** (Botanical name: Curcuma longa)

the yellow pigment in the root of the Turmeric plant which is used in Indian natural medicine (*Ayurveda*) since thousands of years. Scientifically validated, inter alia, at the University of Colorado.

Recommended daily **dosage** up to 800 mg.

In general, to counteract digestive disorders (such as indigestion, stomach pain, gas, bloating, heartburn, nausea, vomiting, belching.) naturally, center piece of this process are **probiotics** (as mentioned above) – speak: a set of 'good bacteria' in form of 'friendly' live microorganisms in the gut – to basically ward off inflammation in your intestines.

One of the best sources for probiotics is, inter alia, non-pasteurized

- ***Sauerkraut***

(*pasteurized* sauerkraut kills active/good bacteria!)

Sources for probiotics are further the fermented milk called

- ***Kefir***

Just as

- ***Natto*** (fermented soybeans)

And

- ***Yogurt***

containing the 'good' bacteria *Lactobacillus bulgaricus* and *Streptococcus thermophilus,* responsible for a healthy balance in the gut. (Read the label to make sure it contains the right bacteria.)

Based on research and scientific validation, respectively at, inter alia, *Johns Hopkins University*, the University *of Bologna* in Italy and the *University of North Carolina* which additionally recommend animal based polyunsaturated

- ***Omega-3***

from animals such as *fish oil* with a daily recommended **dosage** of 1000 mg (1 g) and daily 1000 IU of

- ***Vitamin D***

which helps your body to produce more than 200 antimicrobial peptides to fight all kinds of infections. A daily walk in the sunshine (preferably some 15 minutes at noon) is recommended or orally up to 2000 IU.

In this respect, research at the *University of Granada* in Spain suggests a combination of omega-3 and the naturally occurring flavonoid

- *Quercetin*

which is abundant in **apples**, or which you can get from supplements with a recommended **dosage** of up to 400 mg daily.

Well underestimated is the health value of

- *Asparagus* (Botanical name: Asparagus officinalis)

as an antioxidant to support our biological system and as a 'super food' to challenge chronic disease, including – colon-, heart-, prostate-, breast-, lung-, and other cancers. According to the *University of California* in Los Angeles *(UCLA)*.

Similar are the findings at *Texas A&M University*, scientifically validated by the Foods Standard Agency of the *European Commission,* according to which

- *Dried Plums (Prunes)*

help to maintain an appropriate level of beneficial gut bacteria.

Another encouraging fruit for healthy digestion is

- *Blueberries* (botanical name: Vaccinium angustifolium)

not only because of the antioxidants and vitamins they contain but because of the fiber. Based on research at the *USDA Human Nutrition Center,* the *University of North Carolina,* and the *University of Bologna* in Italy.

According to research at the *American Herbalist Guild* in Halifax, VA, also a daily cup of

- *Peppermint* (Botanical name: Mentha piperita)
  &
- *Elderflower* (Botanical name: Sambucus nigra L.)
  tea can reduce digestive disorder because of its antimicrobial power.

Based on the competence of same *American Herbalist Guild*, also following herbs may help with digestive disorders:

- **Basil** (Botanical name: Ocimum basilicum)
  with a recommended daily **dosage** of up to 500 mg,
- **Thyme** (Botanical name: Thymus vulgaris)
  with a recommended daily **dosage** of up to 600 mg 3 times,
- **Sage** (Botanical name: Salvia officinalis)
  with a recommended daily **dosage** of 150 mg,
  and the aromatic herb
- **Fennel** (Botanical name: Foeniculum vulgare)
  with a recommended daily **dosage** of 3-times up to 500 mg

Similar results have been achieved with a cup of

- **Rosemary** (Botanical name: Rosmarinus officinalis)

Tea – according to the *American Herbalist Guild* in cooperation with the *National Institute of Medical Herbalists* in the UK.

Also, deglycyrrhizinated

- **Licorice root** (Botanical name: Glycyrrhiza glabra)

may help, according to the *Kellman Center for Progressive Medicine* in New York City.

Recommended **dosage** 500 mg 30 minutes before each meal.

Based on the same source of scientific validation, you may fight

- **Gastro Esophageal Reflux Disease (GERD)**
  with 1000 mcg *Vitamin B-12* plus 800 mcg of *folic acid* daily;
- **Ulcers**
  with 800 mcg folic acid daily twice, 500 mg of *licorice root* half an hour before meals, and 2 g of the herb *goldenseal* twice daily;
- **Heartburn**
  with 4 g of the amino acid *L-Glutamine* and again, 500 mg of *licorice root* half an hour before meals, and 1000 mg of *mastic gum* from the sap of Mediterranean pistachio trees;

- **Irritable Bowel Syndrome (IBS)**
  as the manifold cause behind constipation and diarrhea, and which you may relieve with (alternatively) *ginger/lemon balm/peppermint tea* to reduce gas;

- **Crohn's Disease**
  responsible for, inter alia, fever, bloody bowel movements, rectal bleeding, and above all abdominal pain,
  with daily 800 mcg *folic acid*, 500 mg of *licorice root* 30 minutes before meals, 2000 mg of omega-3 fish or flax seed oil 3 times per day, 2 g of the bioflavonoid *quercetin*, 4 g of the amino acid *L-glutamine*, plus 2 g of the herb *goldenseal* twice a day.

Based on research at *Keio University* in Tokyo, Japan, Japanese herbal medicines are recommended for good digestion, such as

- **Dai-Kenchu-to**

a herbal blend of **ginseng, ginger,** and **zanthoxylum,** used also for diarrhea, and

- **Rikkunshi-to**

a blend of 8 crude herbs which is also administered in the U.S. for gastrointestinal distress in cancer patients at, inter alia, *Cleveland Clinic* in Cleveland, OH.

No recommended daily **dosage** for both.

Also,

- **Mediterranean Diet**

is an optimal basis for digestive regulation, according to research at the *University of Bologna*, Italy, because it includes fiber-rich fruits, vegetables, and legumes.

>>><<<

See also chapters
CONSTIPATION, IMMUNITY WEAKNESS,
NAUSEA & VOMITING, TOXICATION

ENERGY LOSS

According to the *Institute for Cancer Research* in New York,

- ***Vitamin A***

is an excellent choice, with a recommended ***dosage*** of up to 10,000 I.U.

- ***Vitamin B-12***

is suggested as a result of the medically famous *Framingham Heart Study* in Framingham, MA.

Recommended daily ***dosage*** up to 1000 mcg; either as a supplement or red meat in your diet.

Also, to support your energy (and counter muscle loss) take

- ***Alpha Lipoic Acid (ALA)***

based on research going back to the 1950s at, inter alia, the *University of Texas* in Austin, TX.

Recommended ***dosage*** 300 mg 2 times daily.

Another 'revolutionary' nutrient is

- ***Procaine HCI***

Composed as a blend of certain molecules and B vitamins, it was developed by French scientists and refined by Romanian doctor Ana Aslan for, inter alia, energy support, cell detoxification, is also a strong power for mental focus, memory enhancement and mood lifting.

For daily ***dosage*** see label.

FATIGUE

Fatigue is a very controversial health problem insofar, as there is no scientific proof yet, if it is a physical or a psychosomatic problem.

In fact, according to – inter alia – the *Center for Effective CFS/Fibromyalgia Therapies* in Annapolis, MD, fatigue can be caused by many metabolic and medical conditions such as, inter alia, hypoglycemia (low blood sugar), depression, insomnia, memory problems, anemia, heart disease, thyroid problems, hormone (estrogen, testosterone) deficiencies – and cancer.

Conventional treatment of cancer such as chemotherapy and radiation challenges the body's biological balance in an especially dramatic way.

One of your body's reactions in this case is fatigue by impairing the adrenal glands, which gives energy and endurance. These unnatural anti-cancer modalities are a heavy toll on your body's natural energy and virtue in a very debilitating way, which can last even years after conventional cancer treatment ended. Validated, inter alia, by research at renowned *Moffitt Cancer Center* in the U.S.

Cancer-related fatigue can also be caused by, e.g., impairment of blood circulation and blood clotting – consequence of cancer treatment side effects such as, inter alia, malnutrition and somatophobic medications. According to research at, inter alia, the *University of Granada* in Spain, depression and *pain* increase *fatigue* – one more of an example how systematically interwoven man as an *ecosystem* is.

Another potential pathway for cancer related fatigue is stress caused by the disease, as demonstrated in a study elaborated at *Ohio State University* Institute of Behavioral Medicine.

While synthetic-chemical medications may not be advisable for counterbalancing cancer treatment related fatigue, following herbs from in- and outside the Rainforest may help:

- *Maca* (Botanical name: Lepidium meyenii)

This plant, also named "Peruvian ginseng', although it does not belong to the botanical 'Ginseng' family, is a native to the high altitude of the South American Andes, with the potential of, inter alia, relieving fatigue naturally.

Scientifically validated, inter alia, at *Northumbria University* in Newcastle, UK.

Recommended daily **dosage** 750 mg 1-2 times daily.

- **Suma** (Botanical name: Pfaffia paniculata)

The roots of this shrubby vine which is also called 'Brazilian Ginseng', are used for inter alia, fatigue, pain, and inflammation with different causes, including cancer, especially in Brazil and Peru.

In our Western hemisphere scientifically validated at, inter alia, the *Jefferson Medical College* in Philadelphia, PA.

Recommended daily **dosage** 1000 mg (1 g) 2-4 times daily.

Similar the results of 2 other herbs from the Amazon Rainforest

- **Muira puama** (Botanical name: Ptychopetalum olacoides)
  Recommended daily **dosage** 1 cup of decoction
- **Yerba mate** (Botanical name: Ilex paraguayiensis)
  Recommended daily **dosage** 1000-2000 mg (1-2 g)
  and
- **Ginseng** (Botanical name: Panax quinquefolius)
  Recommended daily **dosage** 500 mg

According to research and trials of renowned U.S. *Sloan Kettering Cancer Center*.

Another powerful herb to relieve fatigue is known since more than 3000 years in India, researched at the *University of Michigan* and *CSM Medical University* in India, is

- **Ashwagandha** (Botanical name: Withania somnifera)

Recommended daily **dosage** of 2 times 500 mg.

According to research at the *American Herbalist Guild*, also a daily cup of

- **Peppermint** (Botanical name: Mentha piperita)
  &
- **Elderflower** (Botanical name: Sambucus nigra L.)

taken as a tea can reduce fatigue because of its antimicrobial power.

Also from 5000 years old *Traditional Chinese Medicine* (TCM) we know the herbs

- **Astragalus** (Botanical name: Astragalus membranaceus),

according to the *University of Arizona* in Tucson.

Recommended **dosage** 500 mg daily.

- **Eleutherococcus** (Botanical name: Eleutherococcus senticosus),

is another powerhouse of energy enhancement according to studies at M.D. Anderson Cancer Research Center at the *University of Houston*, TX, the largest cancer research institute worldwide.

Recommended as an oral liquid, for daily **dosage** see label.

According to research at, inter alia, the *University of Exeter*, UK,

- **St. John's Wort** (Botanical name: Hypericum perforatum)

can relieve fatigue.

Recommended **dosage** up to 300 mg daily.

Same is with

- **Galantamine**

derived from the plant Caucasian snowdrop (Botanical name: Galanthus caucasicus), according to research at *Erciyes University Medical School* in Kayseri, Turkey.

Recommended daily **dosage** up to 8 mg.

The amino acid

- **L-Ornithine**

found in our diet of, inter alia, dairy products, eggs, fish, meat, may also help with fatigue, according to research at, inter alia, *Wakayama Medical*

University and *Osaka City University Graduate School of Medicine* in Japan.

Recommended daily **dosage** 1500 mg (1.5 g) 3 times daily.

Another nutrient derived from the amino acid l-arginine is

- **Creatine**

which has been validated by research at *Temple University* in Philadelphia, PA, to be effective in cases of fatigue.

Recommended daily **dosage** 4,000 mg (4 g) 6 times daily.

Or take the Chinese mushroom

- **Cordyceps**

to increase your energy level, according to research at the *University of Arizona* in Tucson.

Recommended daily **dosage** 1500 mg (1.5 g) up to 4 times.

- **Cocoa**

also can relieve fatigue by boosting levels of brain chemical serotonin, as validated by research at the *University of Hull*, UK.

- **Green Tea** (Botanical name: Camellia sinensis)

has not only anti-cancerous properties but, according to research at *Osaka City University* Graduate School of Medicine in Japan, can reduce fatigue.

To be rounded up by

- **Vitamin C**

according to research at the *University of Arizona* in Tucson

Recommended daily **dosage** at least 250 mg.

Plus

- *Vitamin E*

    according to research at the *University of Arizona* in Tucson. Recommended daily *dosage* 800 IU.

    Together with a recommended *dosage* of 200 mcg of

- *Selenium*

    as well as a recommended *dosage* of 100 mg of

- *Co-enzyme Q10*

to produce energy in the body, according to research at, inter alia, the *University of Arizona* in Tucson, the *University of Wisconsin*, the *University of California* at Davis, and *Pacific Western University* in Los Angeles.

The latter validated scientifically also the steroid hormone

- *DHEA* (Dehydroepiandrosterone)

with a recommended daily *dosage* of up to 100 mg for *sleep* maximization up to 8 hours per night for increase of energy.

Another co-enzyme with high reputation is

- *Coenzyme-1* also named *NADH*

(which stands for *N*icotinamide *A*denine *D*inucleotide plus high-energy *H*ydrogen), an antioxidant form of Vitamin B-3 for potent production of energy in the cells.

Researched and validated at *Georgetown University Medical Center* in Washington, D.C.

Recommended daily *dosage* 10 mg & see label for further intake advice.

According to research at *Imperial College* and the *University of London - both London,* UK - fatigue is related to musculoskeletal pain and related to an imbalance of a kind of fat - phospholipids – in the brain. This requires including fatty fish like salmon and white albacore tuna in your diet.

Additionally, the *Robert Wood Johnson Medical School* in Brunswick, NJ, recommends, inter alia,

- **Fish Oil** or alternatively **Primrose Oil**
- **Bilberry** or alternatively **Grape seed** extract

For relieving fatigue resulting from conventional cancer treatment we should also consider

- **Physical Exercise**

in terms of moderate daily aerobic physical activity 20-30 minutes at least 5 days per week, as recommended, inter alia, by the & *Moffitt Cancer Center Research Institute* and research at the *University of Arizona* in Tucson.

This is in line with the policy of *Cooper Aerobics Center* in Dallas, TX, Basically validated, inter alia, by the *National Institute of Aging* in Bethesda, MD.

HAIR LOSS

Some 80% of the U.S. population is affected by hair loss (alopecia), an autoimmune disease which, in most cases, is caused by an inflammation of the immune system, where immune system cells attack hair follicles

Also, hair loss can result from deficiencies of protein and certain minerals, primarily

- *Iron*

according to research at, inter alia, *Cleveland Clinic* in Cleveland, OH – one of most prestigious clinics in the U.S. - and the *University of Portsmouth* in Portsmouth, UK.

As well as of

- *Zinc*

Scientifically validated at, inter alia, *Jagiellonian University* in Krakow, Poland.

To balance these deficiencies, have a blood count first and take supplements accordingly.

In many cases alopecia is caused as a side effect of prescription drugs such as anti-depressants, cholesterol-lowering and hypertension drugs, chemical blood thinners, arthritis drugs, chemical painkillers – and those of conventional cancer treatment.

As far as the latter is concerned, hair loss is induced primarily by cytotoxic **chemotherapy** drugs like *Cyclophosphamide*. (Dependent on the dosage, the loss is 20% up to 100 %.). Similar results are seen with *Doxorubicin* and *Methotrexate*.

However, the good news is that, as long as hair *follicles* are still alive, a balanced natural diet with the appropriate building blocks of protein and other essential nutrients can spur hair growth. Inter alia, with vitamins C, D, E, and B-7 (Biotin):

- **Biotin** (Vitamin B-7)

as scientifically validated at the *University of Nebraska* in Lincoln, NE.

Recommended daily **dosage** up to 7,500 mcg daily.

- **Vitamin C**

according to *Kyungpook National University* in South Korea.
Recommended **dosage** up to 500 mg twice daily.

- **Vitamin D**

according to research at, inter alia, the *University of Texas* and *MD Anderson Cancer Center,* both in Houston, TX, *Tel-Aviv University* in Israel, as well as *Marselisborg Hospital* in Aarhus, Denmark.

For appropriate **dosage** prefer 20 minutes of moderate sun exposure, if possible.

As far as

- **Vitamin E**

is concerned, this is based on first ever scientific findings, elaborated at the *Science University* in Malaysia.

Recommended daily **dosage up** to 800 IU.

Another set of natural substances supporting hair growth, at least **topically**, are following herbs in form of **essential oils**, such as

- **Lavender** (Botanical name: Lavendula angustifolia)
- **Rosemary** (Botanical name: Rosmarinus officinalis)
- **Cedar wood** (Botanical name: Cedrus atlantica)
- **Thyme** (Botanical name: Thymus vulgaris)

according to *Aberdeen Royal Infirmary* in Scotland Al-Fateh University in Tripoli, Libya.

As well as

- **Yellow Mountain Laurel** (Botanical name: Kalmia latifolia) root extract, according to *Daejeon University*, South Korea.

  Recommended daily **dosage:** decoction with 10-20 drops 2-3 times daily.

And

- **Super Oxide Dismutase (SOD)** enzyme

  According to research at *Baylor College of Medicine*, Houston, TX.

  Recommended daily **dosage** 250 mg.

Similar positive results are reported about **topical** application of

- **Omega-3**

 rich fish oils according to the *International Oceanic Association of Aquatics and Marine Life.*

Recommended daily **dosage** 1000 mg.

Additionally, you may consider the sulfuric amino acid

- **L-Cysteine**

 according to scientific validation at *PATH Medical Center* in New York.

Recommended daily **dosage** 5000 mg (5 g).

Also eating chili peppers containing

- **Cayenne (Capsicum)**
  which makes chili peppers spicy,
  together with
- **Soy Isoflavones**

are helpful (the latter to be found in soy beans), based on research at *Nagoya City University* and *Kumamoto University*, both in Japan

You can finally also consider a hair transplant; however, it is the opinion of the author trying the natural way as recommended above, first.

HEADACHES

Certain cancer drugs and radiation therapies with an impact on the central nervous system can cause severe headaches.

If this is treated with synthetic medication (painkillers) more than twice a week, stomach upset and other side effects are the consequence, according to research at, inter alia, the *State University of New York* in Brooklyn. Validated by the *National Headache Foundation* in Chicago.

Based on these findings, and scientifically validated also by the *New England Center for Headache* in Stamfort, CT, following key nutrients and other natural modalities are recommended to relieve headaches:

- **Magnesium** 400 mg/day.
- **Vitamin B-2** 400 mg per day for 2-3 months.
- **Lecithin** 200 mg per day.
- **Fish** or **Flaxseed Oil** rich in omega-3 fatty acids, 15 grams per day.
  Also, 125 mg of dried
- **Feverfew** (Botanical name: Tanacetum parthenium L.)

 may help based on the same source of research.

The most commonly used natural remedy for headaches since ancient times, however, is certainly the bark of

- **White Willow** (Botanical name: Salix alba)

according to research at, inter alia, the *University of Maryland*.

For recommended daily **dosage** see label.

Based on the findings at the *Neurological Clinic at Christian-Albrechts University* in Kiel, Germany, 1000 mg of

- **Peppermint Oil**

applied to the forehead is more effective than the equivalent of chemically synthetic Acetaminophen (2 tablets Tylenol) – and without known side effects.

HOT FLASHES

Hot Flashes, not to be misunderstood as 'fever', are a well known phenomenon (side effect) of menopause as a sudden rush of heat, due to change of diameter of blood vessels near skin – rising skin temperature, especially on the upper body and face.

The same happens as a consequence of radiation or when certain chemotherapy drugs damage ovaries with a sudden rush of heat, which can lead also to higher blood pressure (up to 10 points systolic/diastolic) – according to research at *Weill Cornell Medical College* and *Presbyterian Hospital* in New York City.

While hot flashes, primarily, are felt inconvenient, they may also have a negative impact on the brain function of the respective patient, according to the *University of Pittsburgh School of Medicine* in Pennsylvania.

To relieve hot flashes, you may refrain from unfavorable lifestyle issues like smoking, spicy foods, caffeine and large meals, as well as saunas and hot tubs.

Above all, avoid Hormone Replacement Therapy (HRT) some oncologists recommend despite the risk of dramatic side effects. One of the risks is developing breast cancer. Scientifically validated by, inter alia, the *Cancer Prevention Institute of California* (former Northern *California Cancer Center*), the *Harbor-UCLA Medical Center* in Los Angeles and the *Elmhurst Hospital Center* in New York. Also lung cancer, according to the *Oregan Health and Science University* and the *Harbor-UCLA Medical Center* in Torrance, CA.

Because of that, instead of conventional HRT you may apply *Phytoestrogens* (*isoflavones* - natural substances in certain plant foods) like

- *Soy*

according to research at, inter alia, the *University of Minnesota* in St. Paul, Tufts *University School of Medicine* and *University of Montana* in Missoula, and *Griffith University School of Medicine* in Australia.

Validated by the *North American Menopause Society,* by recommending also

- **Black Cohosh** (Botanical name: Actaea racemosa)

Recommended daily **dosage** up to 200 mg.

Another recommendation comes from a small pilot study carried out at Mayo *Breast Clinic* at renowned *Mayo Clinic* in Rochester, MN, according to which

- **Flaxseed** (Botanical name: Linum usitatissimum)

as a rich source of Omega-3 polyunsaturated fatty acids may relieve hot flashes successfully.

Recommended daily **dosage** 1000 mg.

You may additionally consider e.g.

- **Pycnogenol**

a pine bark substance from Sothern France, according to research at, inter alia, the *Keiju Medical Center* in Japan.

Recommended daily **dosage** 150 mg.

According to research at, inter alia, *Stanford University* in California,

- **Acupuncture**

shows some promise for hot flashes, although there is still more scientific evidence needed.

IMMUNITY WEAKNESS

Our immune system is the most powerful defense against anything which may harm our body. Therefore, it is – yes – *vital* to strengthen the immune system by all means.

This is especially important in case of conventional cancer treatment which weakens the immune system dramatically – surgery, chemotherapy and radiation alike. (E.g., radiation diminishes white blood cells.) Additionally to the fact that cancer impairs immunity in general, as scientifically validated at, inter alia, *Chicago University*.

However, it is a myth to believe that the immune system can be supported effectively with a so called synthetic, drug-based *immunotherapy*. Chemical drugs weaken the immune system even more – a vicious cycle.

This fact has been scientifically validated, inter alia, by Drs. Beutler, Hoffmann and Steinman who were granted the Nobel Prize in Physiology in 2011 for their discoveries concerning the activation of innate immunity. Scientifically validated only recently by research at the *University of Michigan,* according to which most patients receiving this kind of treatment 'do not respond'.

To support the immune system naturally instead,

● *Antioxidants*

are very important, according to an innovative study carried out at the *University of Texas Health Science Center* in San Antonio, TX, in cooperation with the *Scripps Research Institute* in Jupiter, Florida – with special reference to **Vitamin C** nutrients.

Based on the fact that, while a healthy vitamin C level in the body should be in the range of 61-80 micromol/L, cancer pushes it down to less than half.

In fact, some 80 years ago, in 1937, Dr. Albert Szent-Gyorgyi has been awarded to Nobel Prize in physiology for his research on vitamin C with special reference to enhancing the immune system. A nutrient available in small amounts in certain plant foods like **orange juice**, according to research at the *University of Granada* in Spain.

Similar are the findings with 250 grams of

- **Blueberries** (Botanical name: Vaccinium angustifolium)

powder boosting the activity on NKCs, according to research at the *Appalachian State University* in Boone, N.C.

Unlike chemotherapy which does not kill *all* cancer cells (that's why we are speaking of 'remission' instead of a cancer cure) NKC's can kill *all* cancer cells. Scientifically validated, inter alia, at the *St. Gerardo Hospital* in Milan, Italy.

Another important vitamin for strong immunity support is

- **Vitamin D**

based on research at, inter alia, the *University of Ulster* in Coleraine, UK, and the *University of Copenhagen* in Denmark.

This is achieved preferably from moderate sun exposure on our skin, or a **dosage** of 2000 IU daily in supplements.

Equally innovative is the finding at the *University of Missouri* in Columbia, MO, according to which

- **Resveratrol**

a polyphenol substance in red grapes and red wine supports also the immunity. Scientifically validated by the *Linus Pauling Institute* at *Oregon State University* in Corvallis. (Named after Dr. Lines Pauling, 2 times Nobel Prize laureate and founder of the *Orthomolecular Medicine* in the 1960s.)

Vice-versa, there is a complex negative influence of *malnutrition* on *infection* and *immunity* according to the *London School of Hygiene & Tropical Medicine,* UK, and the *Max Planck Institute for Infection Biology,* Germany.

A well reputed substance to strengthen the immune system is also

- **Papain**

the enzyme found in the fruit, root, and leaves of **papaya**, based on research at the *University of Maryland.*

Another 'revolutionary' nutrient is

- **Procaine HCI**

Composed as a blend of certain molecules and B vitamins, it was developed by French scientists and refined by Romanian doctor Ana Aslan for, inter alia, immunity support, cell detoxification, is also a strong power for mental focus, memory enhancement and mood lifting.

For daily **dosage** see label.

Similar 'revolutionary' is a product on the natural health market called

- **EpiCor**

containing a complexity of vitamins, minerals, phenolics, and phytosterols, including magnesium, zinc, potassium, calcium, B-vitamins. Scientifically validated, inter alia, the *Medical College of Virginia* in Richmond, VA.

Also in this case, for daily **dosage** see label.

In herbal terms, the probably best remedy to support immunity is an ancient Chinese herb by the name of *Huang qi,* which we know today as

- **Astragalus** (Botanical name: Astragalus membranaceus)

which fights also cancer.

Recommended daily **dosage** 500 mg daily.

Also very important for stabilizing the immune system is

- **Aloe arborescens & Aloe vera**

as these 2 types of herbs of the same family release substances from certain white blood cells originating in the bone marrow - which activate natural killer cells (NKCs) and kill cancer cells by secreting cytotoxic enzymes. Scientifically validated at, inter alia, the *Dana-Farber Cancer Institute* in Boston.

To support your immunity, according to research at, inter alia, the *University of Michigan* and the *CSM Medical University* in India, also the herb

- **Ashwagandha** (Botanical name: Withania somnifera)

has an excellent reputation, with special reference to chemotherapy and radiation.

Recommended daily **dosage** 2 times 500 mg daily.

When talking about nutrients to strengthen the immune system, we should also consider one specific herb, sometimes called the best-kept health miracle in the world, and this is

- **Curcumin** (Botanical name: Curcuma longa)

the yellow pigment in the root of the Turmeric plant which is used in Indian natural medicine (*Ayurveda*) since thousands of years. Scientifically validated, inter alia, at the University of Colorado.

Recommended daily **dosage** 800 mg.

One of the most powerful immunity supporters and cancer fighters is the trace mineral

- **Selenium**

according to research at, inter alia, the *University of Copenhagen* in Denmark.

With a recommended daily **dosage** of 200 mcg and which is naturally found in, inter alia, vegetables of the 'cabbage family', according to research at, inter alia, *Johns Hopkins University*.

Similar is the situation with the level of

- **Copper**

in your blood. Most Americans are deficient of copper. This is responsible for, inter alia, poor sleep. To balance it, the recommended **dosage** is 900 micrograms per day, according to research at the *University of Eastern Finland*.

Scientifically validated by the *Linus Pauling Institute* at *Oregon State University*. (Please note again: Dr. Linus Pauling is a 2-time Nobel Prize laureate and founder of the *Orthomolecular Medicine*.)

While most fruits and vegetables are low in copper, following foods are especially rich in copper: beef liver (more than 4,000 micrograms per 1 oz.) and oyster meat (more than 1500 micrograms per 1 oz.), and also nuts as well as mushrooms.

A link has been found between *immunity* and *anxiety*, based on research at *Columbia University* and *Rockefeller University*, both based in New York City.

INCONTINENCE

Around 50 million people worldwide, and according to *Harvard University* research, some 25 million adults in the U.S. alone are incontinent, i.e. they are losing urine and/or feces unintended. Of those, almost a quarter of American women have pelvic floor and sphincter muscles weakening, leading to urinary incontinence in many cases.

There is a higher risk if overweight or having more than one child. On the other hand, urinary incontinence is often the result of cancer surgery, according to *Memorial Sloan Kettering Cancer Center* in New York. Caused, e.g., by increased bladder pressure, damaged sphincter muscle which controls bladder flow, or muscle spasms.

Basically, there are 2 common types of urinary incontinence:

- Stress incontinence,
  mainly in the female sector after physiologic changes of menopause and bladder muscles weakened by child birth; and

- Urge incontinence,
  sudden and uncontrollable, when the bladder contracts on its own.

In many cases, incontinence is also connected with depression – not biologically but psychologically -, according to research at *Iowa College of Medicine* in Iowa City.

However, while *The Adjustable Continence Therapy (ACT)* in terms of an implanted 'balloon', as developed at *Emory University* in Atlanta, GA may seem as a technical solution, it is not the most effective answer. Same seems to be with the intraurethral injection of myoblasts (adult stem cells obtained by means of patient's biopsy) as developed at the *Universidad de Navarra* in Spain.

Not to talk about prescription drugs for incontinence relief, as in many cases incontinence is caused by side effects of (other) drugs, thus adding another drug (with side effects), closing the vicious cycle of kidney weakness.

Even worse, one of the drugs to stop involuntary bladder contractions prescribed over decades has the reputation to cause high blood pressure, heart palpitations, constipation and dry mouth according to research at, inter alia, the Center for Bladder and Pelvic Dysfunction of *University of Minnesota* in Minneapolis.

To minimize this risk, the U.S. Institutes of Health have funded a *Program to Reduce Incontinence by Diet and Exercise* (PRIDE) to reduce the risk of incontinence with appropriate diet and exercise. Co-funded by the *University of California* in San Francisco and the *San Francisco Veterans Affairs Medical Center,* together with *Brown University* in Providence, R.I., the *University of Arkansas* in Little Rock, and the *University of Alabama* in Birmingham.

Also, to improve pelvic muscle strength, according to research at *State University of New York* (SUNY) in Syracuse, NY, and scientifically validated by *The Vitamin D Council* in San Luis Obispo, CA, an appropriate level of

- ● **Vitamin D**

is advisable, with special reference to moderate exposure to sunshine of approximately 20 minutes at noon time, or as a supplement with a recommended **dosage** up to 2000 I.U.

According to research at *Iran University of Medical Sciences* in Teheran, one teaspoon of

- ● **Magnesium Hydroxide**

twice a day can ease urinary urge incontinence.

Regarding herbal remedies, research has been done with an encouraging outcome at the *Medical College of Wisconsin* with respect to the bark of

- ● **Cinnamon** (Botanical name: Cinnamomum cassia)

with 2 times 500 mg daily, and the Indian folk medicine

- ● **Babchi** (Botanical name: Psoralea corylifolia)

to calm and tone bladder, spleen and kidneys, the latter being the most important organs for bladder control. (No recommended **dosage** known.)

As well as the traditional Chinese herb

- **Astragalus** (Botanical name: Astragalus mebranaceus)

which, according to research at the *Chinese University of Hong Kong* and the *Mountainwest Institute of Herbal Sciences* in Salt Lake City, Utah, tones (pelvic) muscle contractibility and nourishes kidneys.

Recommended **dosage** up to 2 times 250 mg (total 500 mg) daily.

Radiation therapy can cause urinary incontinence in prostate cancer patients, according to research at *Shahid Behesti University of Medical Science* in Teheran, Iran, which may be relieved with

- **Curcumin** (botanical name: Curcuma longa)

which may also decrease the risk of secondary cancers because of radiation.

Recommended daily **dosage** up to 800 mg.

- **Physical Exercise**

improves pelvic muscle strength in combination with bladder training is highly recommended, according to the *National Association for Continence* in Spartanburg, S.C., and the *American Physical Therapy Association (APT)*. Validated by the *Rehabilitation Institute of Chicago* and the *Brigham & Women's Hospital* in Boston. With reference to *Kegel* exercises to strengthen the pelvic floor muscles, developed by American gynecologist Arnold Kegel in 1948.

INFECTIONS

According to the *Trust for America's Health (TFAH)*, every year 170,000 Americans die from (newly emerging and re-emerging) infectious diseases. Around 50,000 in hospitals. MRSA (Methicillin-resistant Staphylococcus aureus) has become the 6th leading cause of death in the U.S., with 90,000 fatalities each year.

Although infections are not a direct consequence of cancer and its treatment with highly cytotoxic drugs, it can result indirectly in many cases in side effects of conventional cancer drug treatment – like **stress, depression, anxiety** - America's greatest health problems today – covered also in this guide.

Also, based on mutual research of the *London School of Hygiene & Tropical Medicine,* UK, and the *Max Planck Institute for Infection Biology,* Germany, there is a complex influence of **malnutrition** on infection and immunity.

Not enough, to close this vicious cycle, infections can trigger heart attacks and strokes, as a ten-year study funded by the *British Heart Foundation (BHF)* reveals.

That's why we should also consider **infections** as an indirect side effect in this context.

At first glance, the answer looks simple since we are used to tackle infections since more than 60 years with *antibiotics* as the no. 1 retreat of mainstream medicine when it comes to infections of any kind.

Unfortunately yet, antibiotics not only have many side effects, your body becomes resistant in many cases. Therefore, antibiotics are not the best answer to infections. Rather, we should learn how to tackle it naturally as recommended, inter alia, by the governmental *National Institute for Health and Care Excellence (NICE)* in the UK.

E.g., if you have a food infection or reason to fear food poisoning, add

- *Cilantro*

leaves to your diet as the most potent salmonella killer on earth according to research at the *University of California* in Berkeley. Even twice as potent as the best sold prescription drug on the market.

Similar the antimicrobial power of

- ***Grape Seed***

extract as scientifically validated at the *University of Texas* and the *Garden Healing Clinic* in Vancouver, British Columbia, Canada.

Recommended **dosage** up to 20 drops of the liquid concentrate.

As far as bladder infection is concerned, of which some 20% of women are affected once or repeatedly per year,

- ***Cranberry***

juice has good reputation according to research at, inter alia, *Worcester Polytechnic Institute* in Worcester, MA, with special reference to urinary tract infections (UTI). Scientifically validated at *Harvard University*.

Also,

- ***Cinnamon*** (Botanical name: Cinnamomum verum)

may well ward off infection, according to research at *New York School of Career and Applied Studies,* a division of *Touro College & University System.*

Recommended **dosage** 1000 mg twice daily.

Very encouraging for different kinds of infections, including polyarthritis, Morbus Crohn, Colitis ulcerosa and asthma, etc. is the 'biblical' herb

- ***Boswelllia*** (Botanical name: Boswellia serrata)

according research at the *University of Giessen* in Germany.

Recommended **dosage** 500 mg 2-3 times daily.

Another natural way to fight bacteria is a cup of

- ***Green Tea*** (Botanical name: Camellia sinensis)

containing 200 mg of **catechins.**

Based on research at *Pace University* in New York, the *University of Illinois* in Chicago, *Alexandria University* in Egypt and the *National Institute of Chemistry* in Ljubliana, Slovenia.

And check your level on following two minerals in your blood:

- ### *Copper*

Most Americans are deficient of copper which may trigger also poor sleep – according to research at the *University of Eastern Finland*.

Scientifically validated by the *Linus Pauling Institute* at *Oregon State University*. (Please note: Dr. Linus Pauling is a 2-time Nobel Prize laureate and founder of the *Orthomolecular Medicine*.)

Recommended **dosage** is 900 micrograms per day.

While most fruits and vegetables are low in copper, following foods are especially rich in copper: beef liver (more than 4,000 micrograms per 1 oz.) and oyster meat (more than 1500 micrograms per 1 oz.), and also nuts (almonds and cashew), as well as mushrooms.

- ### *Zinc*

not only supports the immune system in general but activates those T cells which are conquering viruses and bacteria – according to research at, inter alia, the *University of Florida*.

Recommended daily **dosage** up to 50 mg.

Even most dangerous and deadly MRSA bacteria can be destroyed by certain

- ### *Essential Oils*

i.e., substances found in aromatic plants to avoid infection. According to research at the *University of Manchester*, UK.

INFLAMMATION

Inflammation, derived from the Latin word *inflammo* (meaning "I ignite") is like a phenomenon in geopolitics: the fight against damaged cells and pathogenic 'intruders', and the start of a healing process after. In this respect, inflammation is the body's first defense against infection and part of our body's immune response, accordingly.

Since our body is systemic, any of the multibillions of cells in our body can become inflamed.

This is especially true for cancer, a phenomenon detected already 150 years ago by pathologist Rudolf Virchow for whom cancer was 'a wound that doesn't heal.'

E.g., according to a most recent study elaborated at *Arizona State University*, inflammation is a major trigger of colon cancer metastases.

When it comes to conventional oncologic cancer treatment, the chance of inflammation is even greater, since the chemicals for chemotherapy are the most toxic ones on the market, and radiation being no less dangerous.

Schizophrenically, not only can chemotherapy and radiation cause inflammation – even pre-existing inflammation can support the development of cancer. According to the Charles F. Schmidt College of Medicine at *Florida Atlantic University*, and validated by the U.S. *National Cancer Institute* and the *National Center for Research Resources of the National Institutes of Health*.

Also, it is important to understand that not only are inflammation and **pain** strongly interrelated from a biochemical point of view – those herbs mentioned in the chapter *Pain* are highly appropriate also for *inflammation*. Such as:

- **Aloe Vera** (Botanical name: Aloe vera L.)
- **Amor Seco** (Botanical name: Desmodium adscendens)
- **Anamu** (Botanical name: Petiveria alliacea)
- **Andiroba** (Botanical name: Carapa guianensis)
- **Arnica** (Botanical name: Arnica Montana)
- **Bromelain** (enzyme of pineapples)
- **Catuaba** (Botanical name: Erythroxylum catuaba)

- **Chuchuhuasi** (Botanical name: Maytenus krukovii)
- **Curcumin** (Botanical name: Curcuma longa)
- **Devil's Claw** (Botanical name: Harpagophytum procumbens)
- **Ginger** (Botanical name: Zingiber officinalis)
- **Suma** (Botanical name: Pfaffia paniculata)
- **Tayuya** (Botanical name: Cayaponia tayuya)
- **Willow** (Botanical name: Salix alba)

The same is with

- **Turmeric** (Botanical name: Curcuma longa)

as a relative of **ginger.** It has a 4,000 years old reputation in Indian *Ayurvedic* medicine and *Traditional Chinese Medicine (TCM)* to fight inflammation – nowadays scientifically validated at, inter alia, the *University of Maryland, Tel Aviv University*'s School of Public Health in Israel, and *Memorial Sloan Kettering Cancer Center* in New York.

Recommended daily **dosage** up to 800 mg.

The gum resin of

- **Boswellia** (Botanical name: Boswellia serrata)

also called **Frankincense** in *Ayurvedic* medicine, is helpful in cases of inflammation, according to research at *Long Island University* and scientifically validated by *Memorial Sloan Kettering Cancer Center,* both New York.

Recommended daily **dosage** 500 mg 2-3 times daily.

- **Ashwagandha** (Botanical name: Withania somnifera)

is another important herb with anti-inflammatory impact, according to research at the *University of Michigan* and *CSM Medical University* in India – home country of *Ayurvedic* medicine. Scientifically validated by *Memorial Sloan Kettering Cancer Center* in New York.

Recommended daily **dosage** 2 times 500 mg.

As well as

- **Sage** (Botanical name: Salvia officinalis)

according to research at *Metropolitan State University* in Denver, CO.

Recommended daily **dosage** 150 mg.

Similar results have been achieved with

- **Ginkgo** (Botanical name: Ginkgo biloba)

according to research at *Glasgow Caledonian University* in the UK. Scientifically validated at, inter alia, *Memorial Sloan Kettering Cancer Center.*

Recommended daily **dosage** 60 mg twice daily.

Also

- **Ginseng** (Botanical name: Panax ginseng)

has an excellent reputation to fight inflammation as a kind of *nature's anti-inflammatory*, not only in Asian traditional medicines, but also scientifically validated at, inter alia, the *University of Hong Kong.*

Recommended daily **dosage** up to 500 mg.

Other nutrients are:

- **Resveratrol**

is a polyphenol produced by certain plants, naturally, such as, inter alia, berries and red grapes as a kind of 'immunity' to ward off bacteria and fungi.

According to research at the *University of Buffalo*, the *University of Glasgow*, UK, and the *University of Singapore,* this biochemical background gives this natural substance the power to also ward off inflammation in humans. Cancer included.

Therefore, it is recommended to consume these specific plants and their derivates (including red wine) as an anti-inflammatory measure – with special reference to cancer.

The juice of another berry with ant-inflammatory (and anti-pain) power named

- *Acai*

has been scientifically validated at, inter alia, the *University of Arkansas, Shanghai Institute of Pharmaceutical Industry*, and *AIBMR Life Science, Inc.* It is in fact a 'relative' of red grapes (red wine) as its anti-inflammatory power is based on *anthocyanins*, i.e. pigments also found in red wine.

Also polyphenol- and antioxidant-rich juice of

- *Pomegranate* (Botanical name: Punica granata)

has been found against inflammation based on research at the *University of South Carolina* and *Case Western Reserve University* in Cleveland, OH. Scientifically validated at, inter alia, Memorial *Sloan Kettering Cancer Center*.

Recommended daily *dosage* 1 tbsp.

- *Tart Cherries* (Botanical name: Prunus cerasus)

may equally reduce chronic inflammation, according to *Oregon Health & Science University*, the *Baylor Research Institute* (for medical professionals) in Dallas, TX and the *University of Pennsylvania*.

Recommended daily *dosage* up to 3 times 250 mg each.

Similar positive results have been achieved with

- *Pycnogenol*

a French maritime pine bark substance based on scientific findings of the national Italian *Research Institute on Food and Nutrition* in Rome, Italy.

Recommended daily *dosage* up to 2 times 100 mg.

Another exotic remedy against inflammation, validated at the *Sutter Center for Integrative Health* in Davis, CA, is the Chinese mushroom

- ***Reishi***

to support the immune system and fight inflammation.

Recommended daily ***dosage*** twice 600 mg.

Another natural substance to support anti-inflammatory capacity is

- ***Co-enzyme Q10***

with a recommended daily ***dosage*** of up to 2 times 200 mg.

Also,

- ***Mediterranean Diet***

has an anti-inflammatory effect, based on research at the *University of Cordoba* in Spain, as well as at the *Hospital Universitario Reina Sofia de Cordoba* – the hospital of the same University of Cordoba in Spain, as well as the *University of Pennsylvania* and the *Monell Chemical Senses Center,* both in Philadelphia, PA.

With special reference to

- ***Olive Oil***

as a basic component of the Mediterranean Diet. Based on the natural anti-COX activity of oleocanthal from olive oils.

This effect on inflammation is similar to research carried out at Indiana's *University School of Public Health* on

- ***Magnesium***

Recommended daily ***dosage*** up to 500 mg.

According to most recent studies at the *Fred Hutchinson Cancer Research Center,* and validated by *Mayo Clinic,* **weight loss** with **healthy diet** and **exercise**, in combination with

- ***Vitamin D***

supplementation of 2000 IU ***dosage*** can reduce inflammation, better than weight loss alone.

Scientifically validated also at the *University of Missouri* in Columbia, *Kings's College* in London, and the *University of Bonn* in Germany.

Another important vitamin to fight inflammation is

- ● **Vitamin K-1**

according to research at *Tufts University*. Preferably from food, such as pears, celery, carrots, sun-dried tomatoes, black-/blue-/mulberries, etc.

Recommended daily **dosage** 100 mcg.

An exciting new remedy is

- ● **Green Lipped Mussels** (Scientific name: Perna canaliculus)

found in New Zealand, for chronic inflammation. According to research at *RMIT University* in Melbourne, Australia.

Recommended daily **dosage** 500 mg.

Another encouraging study comes from the *Fred Hutchinson Cancer Research Center* in cooperation with the *University of Washington,* both in Seattle, WA, according to which a combination of

- ● **Fish Oil**
- ● **Glucosamine**
  and
- ● **Chondroitin**

has an anti-inflammatory potential.

The benefit for relieving inflammation with marine-derived

- ● **Omega-3**

fatty acids **EPA** (Eicosapentaenoic acid) and **DHA** (Docosahexaenoic acid) has been scientifically validated at the *University of California* in San Diego, CA, the *University of Newcastle* in Callaghan, New South Wales, Australia, and *Zhejiang University in Hangzhou,* China.

Recommended daily **dosage** 1000 mg.

When it comes to nutrition,

- **_Dairy-rich diet_**

may also be helpful to relieve inflammation, according to research at the *University of Tennessee.*

As well as

- **_Asparagus_** (Asparagus officinalis)

Not only as an antioxidant to support our biological system and as a 'super food' to challenge chronic disease, including - colon, heart, prostate, breast, lung, and other – cancers. Also to relieve inflammation. Based on research at the *University of California* in Los Angeles *(UCLA).*

MALNUTRITION

Malnutrition is not only a matter of quantity, i.e. a lack of a certain amount of calories due to, e.g., loss of appetite. It is basically a matter of quality, i.e. eating unhealthy food, thus producing illness and disease, primarily and recurrently.

This has also a complex negative impact on immunity, according to the *London School of Hygiene & Tropical Medicine,* UK, and the Max *Planck Institute for Infection Biology,* Germany.

According to research at *Texas A&M University,* College Station, TX, healthy diet can prevent and protect against several types of cancer. E.g., the tropical fruit **mango** may help preventing breast cancer.

Unfortunately yet, according to a recent poll by the *World Cancer Research Fund* for the *World Cancer Day* on February 4, 2015, half of the population in the UK and other industrialized countries are not aware of the link between healthy diet and cancer.

As an alarming example, the *World Health Organization (WHO)* has only recently launched a scientific report, according to which red and processed meats beyond a daily consumption of 70 grams can cause colorectal cancer with some 34,000 victims every year globally.

So called *Western* diet with red and processed meat plus refined grains and high-fat dairy products could well increase the risk of death for those diagnosed with prostate cancer – scientifically validated, inter alia, by research at *Harvard University.*

Similar findings have been achieved with research at the *IRCCS-Instituto di Ricerche Farmacologiche* in Italy, in terms of endometrial cancer due to the above mentioned Western diet.

Another alarming global meta-study, involving more than 600,000 participants in more than 50 countries worldwide, with almost 200,000 deaths as the result of *sugary drink* consumption has been elaborated only recently at *Tufts University.* (To be sure, according to the U.S. Centers for Disease Control and Prevention – CDC - , 50% of the U.S. population is regular daily consumers of this deadly 'food', with special reference to teenagers and young adults.)

These findings are in line with those of the U.S. *National Cancer Institute,* according to which chances to develop skin cancer are 6 times higher for those with highest soda intake.

However, it is a myth to believe a 'diet' soft drink may be the healthy answer. The artificial sweeteners are well known by research to cause potentially those diseases we know on top of the list of chronic illnesses in this country: heart failure, cancer, diabetes.

In fact, there are almost unlimited examples of nutrients as part of a healthy diet – with special reference to cancer – like *carotenoids* (such as dark green leafy vegetables, carrots, and sweet potatoes) or *healthy fats* (such as avocados, olives, organic eggs, and small cold water fish).

Organic foods are of special reference, with high levels on vitamins, minerals, and other nutrients important for the biological functioning of our bodies. Unfortunately, this is not clearly understood by half of the population in the industrialized world, according to the *World Cancer Research Fund.*

One of the most effective nutrition is definitely

- **Mediterranean Diet**

with extra virgin olive oil to, e.g., lower the risk of breast cancer – according to, inter alia, the *University of Navarra* in Pamplona, Spain. High intake of fruits, vegetables, nuts, legumes, cereals, potatoes, and fish, and fiber all lead to a risk reduction of endometrial cancer by almost 60% – according to the above mentioned Italian IRCCS Institute.

Specifically healthy in context with the Mediterranean Diet are also peanuts and other nuts (as a source of fiber, omega-3, vitamin E) – scientifically validated, inter alia, at *Maastricht University* in the Netherlands   – and also vitamin C in fruits and vegetables – validated by research at the *University of Copenhagen,* Denmark.

Similar the benefit of

- **Vegetarian Diet**

to lower the risks of cancer by up to 45%, according to research at, inter alia, *Loma Linda University* in Loma Linda, CA and *Cancer Research UK* by looking at 20 different types of cancer in Oxford, England.

• Soy Foods

is another important plant-based diet to reduce (breast) cancer recurrence, according to research at *Georgetown University* in Washington, D.C.

Also, at least once per week consumption of

• Cruciferous Vegetables

such as broccoli, kale, cabbage, cauliflower, Brussels sprouts – also called the 'cabbage family' – are very supportive for the whole biological system of your body with the active ingredient *sulforaphane* and a powerful enzyme (myrosinase) to fight cancer and osteoarthritis.

These findings are based on comprehensive research over a time of more than 20 years at *Johns Hopkins University* in Baltimore, MD. Scientifically validated also by, inter alia, the *Dana-Farber Cancer Institute* in Boston, MA.

In this context we may not overlook the power of *fermented cabbage* – well known as

• Sauerkraut

with its anticancer compounds, based on scientific findings at *MTT Agrifood Research Finland* in Jokioinen, Finland.

Similar, dark green leafy vegetables such as spinach and cabbage reduce the risk of developing diabetes - according to research results at the *University of Leicester* in Leicester, England.

Following foods are comprehensively researched to be especially healthy:

• Apples

as a 'miracle fruit' are a very good source of antioxidants to fight free radicals, as well as reducing considerably bad cholesterol LDL enhancing good cholesterol HDL at the same time within 6 months, according to research at *The Florida State University*.

According to *Wageningen University* in Wageningen, Netherlands, apples may even slash the risk of stroke by half.

Even more, the proverbial 'apple a day' may even potentially diminish the risk of developing lung/colon/breast/mouth cancer because of their inherent substance *quercetin*, according to research at *Dana-Farber Cancer Institute* in Boston, MA.

Another specifically healthy fruit is

- **Blueberries** (Botanical name: Vaccinium angustifolium)

with a variety of benefits, including cognitive performance, reducing the risk of high blood pressure, based on research at, inter alia, *Harvard University, Texas Woman's University* in Denton, TX, the *University of East Anglia* in Norwich, England, and potentially the treatment of Parkinson's based on research at *Memorial University of Newfoundland* in St. John's, Canada.

Similar to

- **Cranberries** (Botanical name: Vaccinium macrocarpon)

which, because of the inherent *benzoic acid* may stop the development of lung and colon cancer, as well as leukemia. Based on research at the *University of Rochester* in Rochester, NY. Scientifically validated by the *Dana-Farber Cancer Institute in* Boston, MA.

Oily

- **Fish**

like salmon, herring, trout, mackerel, sardines, anchovies, supports the heart and the nervous system, according to research at the *University of California (UCLA)* in Los Angeles.

- **Sweet Potatoes**

are on top of the list when it comes to containing, inter alia, vitamins A & C, as well as iron, protein and calcium, according to the *Center for Science in the Public Interest,* located in Washington, D.C.

- **Avocados**

are an explicit health food as well, not only because of high contents of vitamins B, E and K, but also because of their high amount of *monounsaturated* fats. (Not to be mixed up with unhealthy *saturated* fats!) Based on research at, inter alia, *Ohio State University.*

• *Peanuts*

are one of the most undervalued foods on this planet. While most of us may eat them 'for fun', researchers at *Vanderbilt University* in Nashville, TN, concluded that a diet high in these legumes can reduce risk of mortality by up to 25%. With special reference to death from cardiovascular disease.

Equally underestimated is the health value of

• *Asparagus* (Botanical name: Asparagus officinalis)

as an antioxidant to support our biological system and as a 'super food' to challenge chronic disease, including - colon, heart, prostate, breast, lung, and other – cancers. Based on research at, inter alia, the *University of California* in Los Angeles *(UCLA).*

Supplemented by any of the many kinds of

• *Onions*

and shallots which, due to their antioxidant and anti-proliferation power, are not only part of the 'health food' family but may specifically have an anticancer effect. Based on research at, inter alia, *Cornell University* in Ithaca, NY.

As well as

• *Garlic*

Its biochemical *allicin* has not only the power to fight cancer but also to treat MRSA, the superbug in hospitals, according to, inter alia, the *Weill Cornell Medical College* in New York, the *Cancer Research UK* in London and the *Weizmann Institute* in Rehovot, Israel, the *Beijing Institute of Cancer Research* in China – and many other renowned medical schools and research organizations worldwide.

However, sometimes less can be more to reduce the risk of cancer (recurrence) by extending

- ● ***Overnight Fasting***

up to 12 hours, according to research at the *University of California* in San Diego.

Could multi-vitamins potentially fill the gap? Not at all, basically for 2 reasons. First, these supplements are, in many cases, not organic and 'whole' but industrially produced extracts. Second, in most cases they contain only a small fraction of what your body needs.

According to the *London School of Hygiene & Tropical Medicine,* UK, and the *Max Planck Institute for Infection Biology,* Germany, there is a complex influence of malnutrition on **infection** and **immunity.**

>>><<<

See also chapters
INFECTIONS, IMMUNITY WEAKNESS

MEMORY DISORDERS

There are many reasons for poor memory like, e.g. Alzheimer's or Dementia. However, in this guide we shall focus pin-pointed directly or indirectly on the consequences of conventional cancer treatment which can last more than 10 years after the treatment was suspended.

Special reference is given to the highly toxic drugs of chemotherapy which lead to manifold adverse effects such as decreased memory capability and so called 'chemo brain' or 'chemo fog', as validated, inter alia, at the *University of California in Los Angeles* (UCLA) and *Trent University* in Canada.

Unfortunately, there is no encouragement involved in most recent cancer drug developments. E.g., a new class of drugs called *BET Inhibitors* may lead to memory loss – according to scientific validation at *The Rockefeller University* in New York City.

Additionally, memory disorders are enhanced by certain nutrient deficiencies such as a lack of

- *Vitamin B-12*

potentially leading to 'brain fog', dizziness or confusion, according to, inter alia, research at *Harvard University*, the *University of Michigan*, and the *Australian National University*.

In this case, a Vitamin B complex including

- *Vitamin B-2, B-6 & B-9 (Folic Acid)*

together with Vitamin B-12 can be even more powerful, according to, inter alia, clinical research at *Boston VA Hospital*.

Also a deficiency of

- *Vitamin D*

can lead to cognitive impairment, as many research papers, including from *Harvard University* and the *University of Exeter* Peninsula Medical School in the UK, reveal.

In fact, Vitamin D is one of nature's 'wonder drugs' for our existence from tip to toe as, inter alia, *Harvard University* researchers verified. Not enough, Vitamin D can boost survival of colon cancer patients according to latest research at *University of Edinburgh* and *Western General Hospital* in the UK.

The deficiency of vitamin D is not only a matter of malnutrition but also because of inadequate regular sun exposure. (If sun rays fall on your skin – any part of the body – it produces Vitamin D.)

In this context, we should also stop the myth that more than 400 IU of daily Vitamin D input may be counterproductive for your health. In fact, according to latest research at *Calgary University* in Canada and *Boston University* Medical School, up to 20,000 IU of Vitamin D are still safe. This may be especially seen in the light that recurrence of cancer is much dependent on Vitamin D deficiency.

As far as *minerals* are concerned, according to recent research at *Yale University,*

- **Magnesium**

is the best choice to fight memory impairment. Although the role of magnesium in this case is known since the middle of last century, new research especially at *Yale University* has validated it scientifically.

Recommended dosage 400 mg daily.

- **Phosphatidylserine (PS)**

a phospholipid membrane component which has been researched at, inter alia, the *New York University* Langone Medical Center, *Johns Hopkins University,* and many other medical institutions, is one of the natural key elements to fight memory disorders in a manifold way.

Recommended daily **dosage** 100 mg.

As another kind of 'revolutionary' natural substance for improving mental alertness and memory,

- **Pycnogenol**

may be considered, the extract of a French maritime pine bark.

By supporting microcirculation in the brain, Pycnogenol may improve certain cognitive functions such as memory, attention-span, mood, concentration, decision-making, and other cognitive functions – scientifically validated, inter alia, by *Chieti-Pescara University* in Italy and *Swinburne University* in Melbourne, Australia.

It should be taken daily and orally, according to, inter alia, recent research at the *University of California* in Los Angeles (UCLA) and the *University of Basel* in Switzerland, scientifically validated also at the *University of Tokyo* and *Memorial Sloan Kettering Cancer Center* in New York.

Recommended **dosage**: 100mg 1-2 times daily.

According to these research institutions, you may also not miss:

- **Green Tea** (Botanical name: Camellia sinensis)

to support cognitive function and improve concentration and learning ability – based on the amino acid L-theanine which is found exclusively in green tea and which triggers natural chemical changes in the brain.

Similar to Green Tea is the effect of 2 cups of (organic)

- **Cocoa** (Botanical name: Theobroma cacao)

flavonols to keep your brain and thinking skills intact, as part of dietary intervention. (Similar to those flavonols also found in tea and certain fruits and vegetables.) Scientifically validated, inter alia, at *Columbia University* Medical Center, and *New York University* in October 2014.

Also helpful, according to the *Human Cognitive Neuroscience Unit* at the *University of Northumbria* in the United Kingdom may be

- **Lemon Balm** (Botanical name: Melissa officinalis)

for better accuracy of attention.

Recommended daily **dosage** 600 mg.

- **Bacopa** (Botanical name: Bacopa monnieri)

Is another choice based on research at the *University of Wollongong* in Australia is an herb historically known for thousands of years, native also to Indian *Ayurveda* natural medicine and *Traditional Chinese Medicine* (TCM). It is also found in wetlands of states in the U.S. south. This herb is

Recommended **dosage** up to 3 times daily 500 mg.

For cognitive decline and neurological disorders, also known for more than 3000 years known in Indian *Ayurvedic* medicine is the herb

- **Ashwagandha** (Botanical name: Withania somnifera)

according to research at, inter alia, the *University of Michigan* and *CSM Medical University* in India. Scientifically validated, inter alia, at *Memorial Sloan Kettering Cancer Center* in New York, the Indian Defence *Institute of Physiology and Allied Sciences,* and *Jamaia Hamdard University,* last 2 institutions located in India's capital Delhi.

Recommended daily **dosage** 2 times 500 mg.

A new and kind of 'revolutionary' finding is about

- **Turmeric** (Botanical name: Curcuma longa)

This root of a perennial plant of the ginger family, which gives curry its yellow color, has an enormous power of memory boosting according to research at, inter alia, the *Monash Asia Institute of Monash University* in Melbourne, Australia. Scientifically validated by, inter alia, *Memorial Sloan Kettering Cancer Center* in New York.

In fact, this research has scientifically validated what the population of India – more than one billion inhabitants – practices since generations: they consume per capita the highest amount of turmeric worldwide and yes, accordingly, have the lowest incidence of cognitive decline on this planet.

Recommended daily **dosage** 800 mg.

The same applies to

- **Curcumin** (Botanical name: Curcuma longa)

the yellow pigment in the root of the Turmeric plant which is used in Indian natural medicine (*Ayurveda*) since thousands of years. Scientifically validated, inter alia, at the *University of Colorado*, the *Swinburne University of Technology* in Melbourne, Australia, and *Selcuk University* in Turkey.

Another 'revolutionary' nutrient is

- **Procaine HCl**

Composed as a blend of certain molecules and B vitamins, it was developed by French scientists and refined by Romanian doctor Ana Aslan for, inter alia, memory enhancement and mental focus, cell detoxification, and mood lifting.

For daily **dosage** see label.

Excellent reputation to relieve anxiety, stress and depression and cognitive decline has the bark of

- **Magnolia** (Botanical name: Magnolia stellata)

according to the *Institute for Traditional Medicine* in Portland, Oregon.

Recommended daily **dosage** 30 mg.

An important herb native to China, where it also has been researched at *Weifang Medical University* in China, but is grown all over the world meanwhile and scientifically validated at, inter alia, *Memorial Sloan Kettering Cancer Center* in New York, is

- **Ginkgo** (Botanical name: Ginkgo biloba)

which supports the cognitive function and increases memory retention.

Recommended **dosage** up to 100 mg daily.

Just to name the 2 most important Rainforest herbs for memory disorders:

- **Guarana** (Botanical name: *Paullinia cupana*)

According to century old traditional evidence, seed and fruit of this creeping shrub native to the Brazilian Amazon region, has been used to enhance memory. This was supported by research in France and Germany already in the 1940s. Nowadays it is scientifically validated at, inter alia, the Brazilian state universities *Universidad Federal da Paraiba* and the *Universidad Federal de Sao Paulo,* and at *Memorial Sloan Kettering Cancer Center* in New York.

Recommended **dosage** 1g-2g 2 to 3 times daily.

In the U.S. today, it is basically used to increase mental alertness.

- **_Samambaia_** (Botanical name: _Polypodium decumanum_)

The rhizome and leaves of this fern to be found in different countries of South America, traditionally used by the indigenous population for different ailments, has been validated scientifically at the _Camilo Jose Cela University_ in Spain for protecting brain cells.

In this context, please note again: if you want to make use of these (and other) herbs, always see that you consider the whole herb and not an extract if possible. To make use of the whole herb best, preferably drink it as a tea or decoction (½ Tsp. per cup of water up to 3 times daily).

Additionally, there are quite some helpful nutrients in our daily diet such as e.g.

- **_Blue-/Black-/Straw-Berries_**

The berries contain neuroactive substances that are effective on the brain – based on, inter alia, research at _Harvard Medical School, Brigham & Women's Hospital,_ and the USDA Agricultural Research Service's Human Nutrition Research Center at _Tufts University._

Not only this, ellagic acid in berries is helpful to detoxify carcinogens as a weapon against cancer recurrence – according to research at, inter alia, _Ohio State University_ in Columbus, OH, and the _University of Georgia_ in Athens, GA (where the author of this book had a teaching and research assignment).

Also

- **_Blackcurrants_**

(at least those grown in New Zealand) improve attention capacity, according to research at the New Zealand Plant & Food Research, in cooperation with _Northumbria University_ in the U.K.

Also appropriate nutrition including broiled or baked (not fried!)

- **Fish**

at least one time weekly which contains **DHA/EPA as an Omega-3** fatty acid as researched, inter alia, at the *University of California in Los Angeles (UCLA)* and the *University of Pittsburgh* School of Medicine. An even better source of Omega-3 is the oil of **Krill** (shrimplike creatures of the Antarctic Ocean).

Not to forget about

- *Walnuts*

which improve cognitive function, according to, inter alia, the *New York State Institute for Basic Research in Developmental Disabilities*.

Beneficial for blood flow to the brain and cognitive function, accordingly, is

- *Beetroot Juice*

based on scientific findings at *Wake Forest University* in North Carolina.

In more general terms, as far as diet is concerned, you may also focus on

- *Mediterranean Diet*

which preserves memory and cognitive capabilities because of the intake of **DHA/EPA Omega-3** fatty acids – according to, inter alia, *Johns Hopkins University, Harvard University*, the *University of Alabama* in Birmingham, AL, the *Mayo Clinic*, and the *University of Athens*, Greece.

This diet includes most healthy – **organic** – nutrients like sesame seed, lignans, fish, plant-based foods (such as fruits, vegetables, nuts, beans, legumes) and, above all, olive oil.

The latter is probably the most important ingredient of Mediterranean diet – with special reference to cognitive function, as elaborated by 2 German universities – *Goethe University* in Frankfurt and *Technical University of Darmstadt* – and, inter alia, *Columbia University* in New York - according to which Mediterranean diet with olive oil may also lower the risk of *breast cancer*.

In this context, we should also not overlook two natural substances that are found in different berries (blueberries, strawberries), peanuts, and in the skin of red grapes – and finally in red wine:

● **Resveratrol**

It has an effect on a part of the brain (hippocampus) important for memory, mood, and learning. This is supported by the U.S. governmental National Institutes of Health, based on research at, inter alia, *Case Western Reserve University*, as well as the *Texas A&M Health Science Center College of Medicine*.

Not enough, according to recent research at the *University of Colorado Cancer Center* in Denver, Resveratrol incorporates the power of natural chemo-prevention of cancer recurrence in general. The same applies to

● **Pterostilbene**

as a natural component of grape skin and red wine as well.

Therefore, don't be surprised to find these 2 'wonder drugs' of nature (a kind of *'fountain of youth')*. under the key words of, inter alia, *inflammation, immune system, weight management*.

Both scientifically researched and validated at, inter alia, the *University of Miami* School of Medicine.

In this context, we should also mention which kind of food *harms* your memory most according to research at the *University of California* in San Diego: *trans fats*.

Additionally to appropriate nutrients, *aerobic*

● **Physical Exercise**

on a regular basis at least 5 times a week for half an hour each should be included. The increased cerebral blood flow due to exercise helps your brain to function better immediately, makes you more focused and supports your memory.

The benefit of exercising for the brain lies specifically with supplying appropriate blood (and oxygen, not to be overlooked) to the brain. Scientifically validated by, inter alia, *Rush University Medical Center* in Chicago, the *University of Kansas Medical Center*, and the *University of Texas Southwestern Medical Center* in Dallas. And only recently again at the *University of Tsukuba* in Japan.

Similar results have been achieved from the famous long-term, i.e. since 1948 population-based study covering the whole town of Framingham,

Massachusetts – validated by *Harvard University* as well as *Brigham & Women's Hospital* in Boston.

To relieve memory disorders with exercise, according to research at the *Georgia Institute of Technology,*

- **Weight Lifting**

may be additionally beneficial.

The positive side effect of exercise lies also with lowering your Body Mass Index (BMI), and a higher cognitive performance, accordingly to research done at *Konkuk University* in Korea, and supported by the Korean Ministry for Health and Wellness.

It has also been scientifically validated by the *Saarland University* in Germany, that a short

- **Nap**

can be very beneficial for brain performance.

Researchers at the *Ruhr University* in Bochum, Germany, also found out about an interesting link between permanent *stress* and mental disorders. This is an interesting example of the *holistic* organization of our body.

And since a cancer diagnosis certainly leads to permanent stress, this phenomenal link between stress and mental disorders is realistic for those diagnosed with cancer. (Please see also chapter on **Stress** in this book.)

MOOD SWINGS

Mood swings are a signal not for a mental illness but an unbalanced phase in life due to, e.g., physical problems or social disturbances. In case of a serious disease, mood swings are a common symptom, which need to be re-balanced before it harms vital organs of the body like the heart.

According to research at the *University of Texas M.D. Anderson Cancer Center* in Houston, TX, the *Fox Chase Cancer Center*, PA and the *University of Pennsylvania*, both in Philadelphia, PA, **emotional well-being** has quite an impact on the outcome of cancer disease.

This problem has been well understood by, e.g., the *American Psychosomatic Society* at their 64th Annual Scientific Meeting, when the *University of Pittsburgh School of Medicine* presented their research. According to this, mood swings may be balanced out with

- **Omega-3**

polyunsaturated fatty acids. Fish is the best source in this situation – based on the findings that the respective blood level of omega-3 fatty acids has an impact on depression, schizophrenia, bipolar disorder, attention deficit, and other psychosomatic issues.

Scientifically validated, inter alia, by British researchers at the *University of Oxford,* the *London Metropolitan University*, and the *Swallownest Court Hospital* in Sheffield, UK.

Another mood improving natural substance is

- **Vitamin D**

evidence-based on findings of *Children's Hospital and Research Center Oakland* and scientifically validated at *Washington University School of Medicine.*

Preferably, vitamin D should be 'tapped' from moderate sunshine insofar, as sunshine falling on your skin (any part of your body) produces vitamin D readily for use by your body. If you do not have this opportunity, make sure that you get vitamin D from dairy and/or supplements.

Recommended daily **dosage** from supplements: 2000 IU.

Similar is the effect of the trace mineral

- **Selenium**

on the mind and emotions, according to the findings of the *U.S. Department of Agriculture's Research Service.*

Recommended daily **dosage** 200 mcg.

Also, when talking about nutrients to regulate mood, we should consider one specific herb, sometimes called a brain supporting miracle from nature, and this is

- **Curcumin** (Botanical name: Curcuma longa)

the yellow pigment in the root of the Turmeric plant, which is used in Indian natural medicine (*Ayurveda*) since thousands of years. Scientifically validated, inter alia, at the *University of Colorado* and *Swinburne University of Technology* in Melbourne, Australia.

Recommended daily **dosage** 800 mg.

Also the herb

- **Black Cohosh** (Botanical name: Actaea racemosa)

is suggested to overcome mood swings –based on research at, inter alia, the *University of Montana* in Missoula, and scientifically validated at, inter alia, *Memorial Sloan Kettering Cancer Center* in New York.

Recommended **dosage** up to 40 mg twice daily.

Another 'revolutionary' nutrient is

- **Procaine HCI**

Composed as a blend of certain molecules and B vitamins, it was developed by French scientists and refined by Romanian doctor Ana Aslan for, inter alia, mood lifting, and cell detoxification. It is also a strong power for mental focus, and memory enhancement. (For daily **dosage** see label.)

You may also consider the amino acid

- ### *L-Tryptophan*

which enhances mood and is converted in to the key neurotransmitter *serotonin* from foods such as bananas, oats, meat, yogurt, milk, chicken, peanuts, dried dates, turkey – based on research at, inter alia, the *University of New South Wales* in Sydney, Australia.

According to research at the *University of Otago*, the oldest university in New Zealand, located in Dunedin,

- ### *Fruits & Vegetables*

support mood, helping to be happier, calmer, and more energetic.

According to similar findings at the *National Autonomous University of Mexico*, certain foods such as strawberries, raspberries, blueberries, cocoa and teas can elevate mood. Validated also by the American Chemical Society.

Another powerful natural substance as a mood enhancer is

- ### *Resveratrol*

to be found, inter alia, in red wine and red grapes –according to research at, inter alia, *Texas A&M University.*

In general,

- ### *Vitamins & Minerals*

are mood enhancing according to *Swansea University* in Swansea, UK.

This implies the necessity of consuming much fruit and vegetables in line with a healthy diet.

Not as a remedy but no less important is aerobic

- ### *Physical Exercise*

at least 20 minutes per week, according to scientific validation at renowned *Johns Hopkins University.*

This way, your brain produces *endorphins, which make* you 'happy' – the natural way. (Refrain from legal and illegal drugs promising the same result!)

>>><<<

See also chapters
ANXIETY, DEPRESSION, STRESS

MUSCLE LOSS

When cancer spreads to the bones (typically in cases of breast, lung, prostate cancer and multiple myeloma), this is not only a potential matter of osteoporosis, it can also weaken muscles, additional to pain, fractures, nerve compressions. For which conventional oncology has no answer yet, according to research at *Indiana University*.

According to research at, inter alia, the *University of Queensland* in Brisbane, Australia,

- ***Omega-3***

polyunsaturated fatty acids derived from fish oil are considered helpful. Validated also by research at *Washington University* in St. Louis, Missouri.

Recommended ***dosage*** up to 1500 mg 2 times daily.

Same researchers in St. Louis also found that

- ***Beetroot Juice***

improves muscle power.

- ***Alpha Lipoic Acid (ALA)***

is an additionally helpful nutrient based on research going back to the 1950s at, inter alia, the *University of Texas* in Austin, TX.

Recommended ***dosage*** 300 mg 2 times daily.

Also,

- ***Vitamin E***

is helpful to build strong muscles, according to research at *Georgia Regents University* in Augusta, GA.

Recommended ***dosage*** up to 1000 IU daily maximum.

As well as a

- *Protein*

-rich diet with, e.g. a cereal breakfast, sandwich or salad for lunch, and meat for dinner.

Based on research at the *University of Texas* in Galveston, *the International Sarcopenia Initiative* and *Hospital Universitario Ramon y Cajal* in Madrid, Spain.

Aerobic physical exercise should support all efforts – with special reference to

- *Stretching*

for building strength and endurance. According to research at, inter alia, *Louisiana State University* in Baton Rouge, *Brigham Young University* in Hawaii, and the *American College of Sports Medicine (ACSM)* in Indianapolis.

A kind of 'exotic' finding comes from the *University of Iowa,* with respect to *ursolic acid* for strengthening muscles, to be found in

- *Apple Peel*

and *tomatidine,* a substance in

- *Green Tomatoes*

NAUSEA & VOMITING

Nausea and vomiting (emesis), besides hair loss, are the unwelcome and dreaded consequences of (highly emetogenic cisplatin-based) chemotherapy and radiation, of which up to 90% of cancer patients are affected. This depends on the type of medication and the duration of treatment.

Yet, it is widely ignored by conventional oncology.

Unlike chemical anti-nausea drugs with their side effects, the herb

- *Ginger* (Botanical name: Zingiber officinale)

derived from the rhizome and consumed as a tea is by far the best natural alternative. Based on research at the University of Michigan, *University of Rochester* in Rochester, NY, and the Royal Hospital for Women in Sydney, Australia and scientifically validated by the *Memorial Sloan Kettering Center* in New York.

Recommended *dosage:* 2-3 cups of tea or up to 1 g powdered Ginger daily.

Additionally, you may consider one or 2 of following 10 Rainforest herbs in alphabetical order (for recommended *dosage* see labels):

- *Artichoke* (Botanical name: Cynara scolymus)
- *Boldo* (Botanical name: Peumus boldus)
- *Carqueia* (Botanical name: Baccharis genistelloides)
- *Fedegoso* (Botanical name: Cassia occidentalis)
- *Gervao* (Botanical name: Startytacheta sp)
- *Guava* (Botanical name: Psidium guajava)
- *Jurubeba* (Botanical name: Solanum paniculatum)
- *Kalanchoe* (Botanical name: Kalanchoe pinnata)
- *Macela* (Botanical name: Achyrocline satureoides)
- *Mullaca* (Botanical name: Physalis angulata)

In terms of food, take

- **Small amounts of food several times daily**
  with
- **Plenty of spring water (no gas)**

As an exotic but, according to the *University of Kentucky Markey Cancer Center* helpful method is the

- **Touch Therapy 'Shin Jyutsu'**

to relieve cancer treatment side effects, especially pain and nausea.

OSTEOPOROSIS

Biological reasons for developing osteoporosis (loss of bone mass and fractures), may be **belly fat** (according to *Harvard University* and *University of Michigan Comprehensive Cancer Center)*, or **high blood pressure**, (according to *St. George's Hospital Medical School* in London), or **depression**, (according to *Max Planck Institute of Psychiatry* in Munich, Germany).

Besides of that *chemotherapy* weakens bone mass and supports osteoporosis. (Scientifically validated at, inter alia, *Indiana University* in Bloomington, IN.

This is especially the case with breast cancer (treated with aromatase inhibitors), and prostate cancer (treated with androgen deprivation and bisphosphonate treatment), according to research and scientific validation at the *Universite de Montreal,* the *Centre Hospitalier de l'Universite de Montreal (CHUM), McMaster University,* the *University of Toronto* and the *University of British Columbia*, all in Canada.

There is a potential impact on the bones also with prostate cancer metastasis due to radiation.

Conventional *bisphosphonate* treatments for enhancing bone density and reducing fracture risk have a negative impact on the bone remodeling cycle. These treatments enhance the risk of atypical fractures, as scientifically validated at top ranked *Hospital for Special Surgery* and *Columbia University* in New York. In other words, while bisphosphonate improve the bone *quantity,* they ruin its *quality.*

Osteoporosis drugs have many other side effects, which, inter alia, can cause even severe vision problems, according to research at *Oregon Health and Science University* in Portland, OR.

Therefore, it is vital, to counterbalance bone loss and treat osteoporosis by appropriate healthy diet – with special consideration of Vitamin D, Calcium, Protein, as well as physical exercise. According to, inter alia, the *International Osteoporosis Foundation, Tufts University* and the *Medical College of Wisconsin* in Milwaukee, WI.

Include in your diet

- ***Vitamin D***

preferably from a vitamin D rich diet such as whole grain cereals, eggs, salmon, tofu, soy yogurt, cod liver oil or mushrooms. Or – if it's appropriate for you – you may exposure of your face and arms to the sun 2 or 3 times a week for 10 minutes.

Another option is to take up to 2000 IU as a supplement, according to research at, inter alia, *Boston University* and *Tufts University,* validated also at *Massachusetts General Hospital* and the *University of Maastricht,* Netherlands. Rounded up with

- ***Calcium***

preferably from calcium rich nutrition as well such as, inter alia, dark green leafy vegetables such as spinach, turnips, kale, broccoli, beet greens and collard greens), non-fat dry milk, skim milk, cheddar cheese, fish (like salmon, oysters, sardines etc.), corn flakes, yogurt, soybeans.

Or take it as a supplement with a recommended daily ***dosage*** of up to 500 mg 3 times daily and together with magnesium for better absorption, according to research at, inter alia, *Tuft's University,* the *Australian Catholic University,* and the *University of* Utah.

How vital indispensable vitamin D and calcium for healthy bones are, has been stressed one more time at the *World Osteoporosis Day* on October 20, 2015, by the *International Osteoporosis Foundation* and Tuft's University *in Boston.*

According to a recent meta-analysis of the U.S. *National Osteoporosis Foundation* involving 8 clinical trials with more than 30,000 participants, supplementation of 1,200 mg calcium and 800 IU of vitamin D per day, reduced the hip fracture risk by no less than 30%.

The importance of calcium and vitamin D-3 (which is important to 'guide' calcium to the bones) has been stressed by research at the *University of Western Sydney Centre for Complementary Research*. Scientifically validated at the *Glendale Memorial Medical Center* for bone health in Glendale, CA.

According to research at *Harvard University* vitamin D is even more important than calcium.

The importance of calcium and vitamin D to reduce bone loss and fractures is also supported by the *International Osteoporosis Foundation* with HQ in Nyon, Switzerland.

With respect to calcium carbonate, which is derived from oyster shells, the *Creighton University Osteoporosis Research Center* in Omaha, Nebraska, recommends up to 1,200 mg daily with food such as low-fat milk, yogurt, and up to 490 mg of cheese.

To help extracting calcium from food, you should add a 'dash' of vinegar – according to research at *Ebetsu University* (*Rakuno Gakuen University*) in Ebetsu, Japan.

Along with a daily **dosage** of 10 mg of

- *Vitamin K-2*

which inhibits loss of calcium from the bones and supports bone density. It is naturally found in asparagus (in fact the no. 1 source) as well as leafy green vegetables such as spinach and iceberg lettuce – according to research at, inter alia, *Harvard University* and the *University of California* in Los Angeles (*UCLA*),.

Another important mineral with regard to bone mineral density is

- *Iron*

with a recommended daily **dosage** of at least 18 mg, according to research at the *University of Arizona,* the *University of Arkansas,* and *Columbia University.*

Similar is the positive results of a recent trial at the *Tahoma Clinic* in Tukwila, WA, with a combo of calcium, vitamin D, vitamin k-2, magnesium, potassium and

- *Strontium*

which is also stimulating the growth of new bone.

Recommended daily **dosage** up to 680 mg.

(Please don't mix up with radioactive *strontium 90*; rather, we are talking about elementary strontium.)

Additionally, up to 500 mg of

- ● **Magnesium**

will maintain the body's calcium level, according to research at, inter alia, *Johns Hopkins University* in Baltimore, MD, the *University of Milan* in Italy and *Loma Linda University* in Loma Linda, CA.

Magnesium is abundantly found in many foods such as, inter alia, spinach, whole grains, beans, peas, nuts, and seeds. According to *Mayo Clinic,* magnesium may be administered also intravenously (IV).

To combine magnesium and calcium is especially helpful for osteoporosis according to the *Silbersee Paracelsus Hospital* in Hannover, Germany.

Up to 3 mg of

- ● **Boron**

is most effective for prevention and treatment of osteoporosis – according to *Grand Forks Human Nutrition Research Center* in Grand Forks, ND.

As well as 5 mg of

- ● **Manganese**

and 50 mg of

- ● **Vitamin B-6**

plus 1 mg of

- ● **Folic Acid** (Vitamin B-9)

are recommended by the *American Holistic Center* in Chicago.

Also,

- ● **Vitamin B-12**

is strongly recommended to balance low bone mineral density, according to research at *Tufts University* in Boston – with a daily **dosage** of 2.4

micrograms. Natural sources of vitamin B-12 are, inter alia, poultry, eggs, salmon, and lean meat.

In addition

- **_Vitamin C_**

helps calcium to reach the bones – with a recommended daily **_dosage_** of 1000 mg or equivalent in vitamin C rich diet, especially fruits and vegetables. According to same research source.

Similar the research results at the _American University of Beirut_, Lebanon, according to which a combo of **_vitamins B/complex, C, E and K_** correlated positively with bone mineral density (BMD).

Vitamins B-6 and K are also stressed for bone building at _Queen's Hospital_ in Burton-on-Trent, Staffordshire, UK.

Also dietary

- **_Silicon_**

found in whole grains (and beer) helps bone formation, and reduces bone loss, according to research at _St. Thomas Hospital_ in London.

Another important mineral for bone density is

- **_Copper_**

of which most Americans are deficient. To balance it, the recommended **_dosage_** is 900 micrograms per day, according to research at the _University of Eastern Finland._

This is also scientifically validated by the _Linus Pauling Institute_ at _Oregon State University_. (Please note: Dr. Linus Pauling is a 2-time Nobel Prize laureate and founder of the _Orthomolecular Medicine_.)

While most fruits and vegetables are low in copper, following foods are especially rich in copper: beef liver (more than 4,000 micrograms per 1 oz.) and oyster meat (more than 1500 micrograms per 1 oz.), and also nuts (almonds and cashew), as well as mushrooms.

Additionally,

● **Phosphorus**

which works together with calcium, is helpful, according to research at *Johns Hopkins University* in Baltimore, MD. Since phosphorus is found in almost any food, such as fish, eggs, dried peas and beans, no supplementation is needed.

According to same research at *Johns Hopkins University*,

● **Potassium**

with a daily **dosage** of 4,700 mg is helpful to decrease calcium excretion. It is found abundantly in foods such as yogurt, tomatoes, spinach, potatoes, whole grains, nuts and seeds, bananas. This is also scientifically validated at the *University of Surrey* in Guildford, Surrey, UK.

Another nutrient to prevent bone loss is

● **Turmeric** (Botanical name: Curcuma longa)

with a recommended daily **dosage** of up to 800 mg, based on research at the *University of Arizona.*

Consider also the nutritional factor

● **Protein**

with, inter alia, salmon as a good source, according to comprehensive research at, inter alia, *Creighton University.*

Especially include protein and isoflavones from

● **Soybeans**

according to research at the *University of Hull* in the UK, scientifically validated by the *International Osteoporosis Foundation.*

Add up to 110 mg of Soy protein which enhances bon-mineral density (BMD) and bone-mineral content (BMC) – according to research at *Tufts University* and validated by research at *Oklahoma State University* in Stillwater, OK (where the author had a teaching and research assignment) and *Loma Linda University* in Loma Linda, CA.

Also, eating **lettuce** is good for stronger bones – based on research at the *University of Bern* in Switzerland.

For bone building they also suggest to include 500 mg daily of

- **Onions**

Similar positive findings were achieved in a study by *Tufts University* and *Boston University* with

- **Carotenoids,**

especially **lycopene**, a phytochemical found in tomatoes and other red fruits/vegetables, which supports bone formation and lowers the risk of fractures. Scientifically validated also at the *University of Toronto* and the calcium research laboratory of *St. Michael's Hospital* in Toronto.

On the other hand, according to research at *Tufts University*, drinking *cola* (and other soft drinks) is counterproductive, as it weakens bone density because of phosphoric acid, lowering the calcium level in the body.

A kind of 'exotic' recommendation comes from Australia's *RMIT University*, according to which

- **Green-lipped mussel** (Scientific name: Perna canaliculus)

a shellfish native to New Zealand, may help with osteoporosis.

Recommended daily **dosage** 1000 mg.

Very helpful is

- **Mediterranean Diet**

for bone protection, according to research at, inter alia, the *Hospital Dr. Joseph Trueta* in Girona, Spain. This diet enhances the concentrations of *osteocalcin* and other bone-formation substances.

This is especially with regard to **fruits, vegetables,** and **dietary fiber** according also to, inter alia, *Tufts University,* and **olive oil** according to research at, inter alia, the *Harokopio University* in Athens, Greece.

And enjoy

- ***Physical Activity***

45 minutes daily according to the *University of Florida* in Gainesville, or at least 30 minutes 2-3 times per week with, e.g., brisk walking, jogging, etc. According to the *National Osteoporosis Foundation* and *Helen Hayes Hospital in* Haverstraw, New York.

Also **gardening** helps according to research at the *University of Arkansas* in Fayetteville, AK.

Similar **weight-bearing exercise** 30 minutes 4 times a week may increase bone density and avoid fragile bones and fractures, also according to research at *Tufts University* and **strength training**, according to the *American Council on Exercise* in San Diego, CA.

However, according to research at *Pennsylvania State University,* **low-weight, high repetition resistance training** increases bone mineral density better than heavy-weight training.

As far as *physical exercise* is concerned, the *YMCA* in Boothbay Harbor, Maine, is applying a specific bone-building program you may want to tap.

Findings on *calcium* and exercise are supported by *Stanford University,* the *Institute for Quality and Efficiency in Health Care* in Cologne, Germany, and the *Royal Australian College of General Practitioners* in Melbourne, Australia.

The importance of *calcium, vitamin D, and exercise* with respect to preventing and overcoming osteoporosis is also stressed by the *Association of Reproductive Health Professionals (ARHP)* in Washington, D.C., based on findings at the *University of Cincinnati* in Cincinnati, OH, and *Creighton University.*

Additionally,

- ***Melatonin***

strengthens bones, according to research at *McGill University* in Montreal, Canada, and the *University of Madrid* in Spain.

PAIN

Pain (Greek 'ponos' - 'body fights back' -, coined by ancient Greek physician and philosopher Hippocrates) is a neurological signal to our brain telling us that there is something wrong in this or that specific part of our body. In this respect, pain is not an illness or disease, but a *symptom* which still ruins our life quality for almost 20% of the U.S. adult population, according to research at *Washington State University* in Spokane.

Although Americans, in international average, get more pharmaceutical medications for pain after surgery, still suffer more pain than others worldwide according to research at the *University Hospital Jena* in Germany.

Even worse, according to research at *Brown University* in Providence, R.I., 26% of American cancer patients get no pain-related therapy at all.

Cancer-related surgery and painful back spasms due to chemotherapy are no exception. This has been scientifically validated at, inter alia, the *University of Rochester Cancer Center* in New York and the *Utah Pain Research Center* in Salt Lake City, UT.

Unfortunately, most cancer patients follow a very harmful procedure to stop pain. Synthetic-chemical drugs – such as, inter alia, transdermal fentanyl, codeine, oral morphine, and oral oxycodone – relieve pain temporarily - with debilitating side effects.

Based on scientific research in the UK, 2000 patients die there each year from side effects of pharmaceutical painkillers (non-steroidal anti-inflammatory inhibitors). Compared with the size of the U.S., this death toll rises to 9000.

According to the *U.S. Centers for Disease Control and Prevention*, the number of death of women because of prescription painkillers has increased five-fold in first decade of this century alone, with almost 50,000 fatalities. Painkillers are the most prescribed drugs in the U.S., followed by cholesterol statins and anti-depressants.

The prescription pain killer *Methadione* increases your risk of death by almost 50%, according to recent research at *Vanderbilt University*. The same problem is with *Acetaminophen*. This is not only the most widely used industrial OTC pain killer globally, but the most underestimated pain drug worldwide – according to research at *Leeds Institute of Rheumatic and Musculoskeletal Medicine in the UK*.

This is why the FDA launched a warning that OTC painkillers (NSAID's) cause a severe risk of heart attack and stroke.

Also, refrain from *opioids* for chronic pain relief. These have debilitating side effects as well, such as foggy brain/mental cloudiness, respiratory problems – and 17,000 deaths due to overdose, according to the U.S. *National Institutes of Health*. According to *Johns Hopkins University* in Baltimore, MD, between 2002 and 2013, the heroin-related death toll quadrupled, with 8,200 deaths in 2013 alone, by almost half a million treatments in 2013.

Similar is the situation with *marijuana* as a pain killer, which has a dramatic effect on the brain, along with other debilitating side effects such as the impairment of memory. Scientifically validated at, inter alia, the *University of East Anglia* in the UK, and the *University of Pompeu Fabra* in Barcelona, Spain.

The fact that some US States and Canada have legalized *cannabis* for medical purposes, with a registry for users established at Canadian *McGill University*, may not be taken as a scientific validation of any kind.

The U.S. Office of National Drug Policy, the U.S. *National Institute of Drug Abuse* and the FDA have launched a dramatic warning about painkillers only recently.

This is especially problematic if cancer is involved, with some 50% of cancer patients experiencing associated pain, as tumors are crushing organs, compressing nerves, and blocking up vessels.

There are 2 types of cancer pain: persistent and temporary. The latter is called *breakthrough pain (BTP)* and occurs in around 40% of cancer cases, appearing acute and lasting up to around one hour with up to 5 episodes daily.

According to the *University of Texas MD Anderson Cancer Center* in Houston, TX, one third of cancer patients are even *undertreated* when it comes to cancer related pain.

That's why according to the internationally renowned *European Pain in Cancer Survey (EPIC)* patients are mostly desperate about this debilitating pain treatment. It has a dramatic impact on daily life performance and social interaction with family, friends, and at workplaces.

40% of pain sufferers in hospices are cancer patients – treated up to 99% with pharmacological pain killers which create even more health problems – premature death potentially included.

Painkillers are the 4th leading cause of premature death in the United States. Not only that: According to Gil Kerlikowske, director of the U.S. Office of National Drug Control Policy, 100 Americans die of drug overdoses each day.

The complexity of our biological system is revealed, when pain combined with depression is leading also to fatigue in cancer patients. This is cientifically validated by the *University of Granada* in Spain.

Not surprisingly, the death rate of painkillers tripled in the US in the last ten years (more than from heroin and cocaine!) – up to more than 15,000 per year, as registered by the U.S. governmental *Centers for Disease Control and Prevention (CDC)*. Narcotics on prescription alone kill 40 citizens per day. CDC Director Dr. Thomas Frieden: *"We are in the midst of an epidemic."*

The fact that these chemicals are recommended on the WHO Model List of Essential Medicines, does not make them better at all.

The most dangerous pain killers are:

- Acetaminophen, with more than 56,000 visits of hospital's Emergency Rooms (ER), 2,600 hospitalizations and 458 deaths due to liver failure per year;
- Acetylsalicylate, with clinically proven frequent gastrointestinal bleedings and perforated ulcers as a consequence;
- Non-steroidal Anti-inflammatory drugs (NSAIDs);
- Cox-2 Inhibitors, with high risk of heart attack.

(These synthetic chemicals are sold by very familiar brand names you have heard about. For details ask your pharmacist.)

If you survive, chances are good you develop long-term side effects like, inter alia, liver failure, cardiovascular problems, kidney failure, gastrointestinal bleedings, and also hearing loss – even in regular, non-overuse cases. Scientifically validated, inter alia, by *Harvard University* in clinical trials with more than 100,000 male and female participants.

According to latest research at *McGill University* more Americans die prematurely from prescription painkillers than cocaine and heroin together. This is due to poisoning part of the nervous system and related side effects. The USA is worldwide #1, followed by Canada #2 – as published in the *American Journal of Public Health*.

Also, prescription painkillers especially for cancer may cause **stroke**, one of the leading causes of premature death in the U.S., according to recent scientific findings at *Aarhus University Hospital* in Aarhus, Denmark.

In a nutshell, the U.S., foremost worldwide in modern medicine and (legally) the most 'drugged' nation in the world, spends most on 'mainstream' medicine globally. Despite of that, it has the lowest life expectancy in the industrialized world.

That leaves us with the question, if there are natural alternatives, without shortening our life expectancy, and without dramatic side effects, at all. YES, there are.

Narcotic painkillers (opioids) like heroin are not included in this terminology, as some believe, taking those 'herbs' for *natural*. Not only have the narcotics a negative effect on, inter alia, brain, heart and breathing (including the possibility of death by immediate stop of breathing), heroin alone is responsible of 3000 deaths in the U.S. per year (including Oscar-winning movie celebrity Philip Seymour Hoffman).

Prescription painkillers and opiods together produce over 20000 deaths per year in the U.S. – more than coming to death by murder and car accidents!

Studies developed at the *University of Chicago* Medical Center show that opiate based pain relievers even support the recurrence of cancer.

Is *marijuana (cannabis)* an option instead? Not at all as, inter alia, *Northwestern University* Feinberg School of Medicine validated in an appropriate trial. Marijuana can lead to severe brain damages, with special reference to memory capabilities, similar to schizophrenia, even years after stopping consumption.

What are the natural alternatives?

Following herbs from in- and outside of the *Rainforest* (the 'biggest natural pharmacy' on our globe) are recommended, scientifically validated, – in fact for both – **pain** and **inflammation.** Like

- **Amor Seco** (Botanical name: Desmodium adscendens)

A weedy perennial herb, aerial parts and dried leaves are used, for, inter alia, pain relief, especially in Brazil, Belize, and the United States. Scientifically validated, inter alia, at the U.S. *Georgetown University* Medical Center.

Recommended **dosage** decoction 1 cup/ ½ Tsp. 1-3 times daily.

- **Anamu** (Botanical name: Petiveria alliacea)

is a perennial herb, which is used as a whole for pain relief in Brazil and Paraguay, and in Cuba even against cancer. Scientifically validated at, inter alia, the *University of Sao Paulo* in Brazil.

Recommended **dosage** decoction 1 cup/ ½ Tsp. 1-3 times daily.

- **Andiroba** (Botanical name: Carapa guianensis)

seed oils, bark and leaves of this tall Amazonian plant – also called *Brazilian Mahogany* – are used as a (topical) pain reliever (especially in Guayana and Brazil), but also for wound healing (again in Guyana).

Scientifically validated, inter alia, at *Columbia University* in New York.

Recommended **dosage** decoction 1 cup/ ½ Tsp. 1-3 times daily.

While the Rainforest herbs should be taken usually orally as a tea or decoction, Andiroba is an exception, as it is applied since many centuries topically only – as an extract of the seed oil of this tall Amazon Rainforest tree.

- **Arnica** (Botanical name: Arnica montana)

A perennial herb and natural non-steroidal anti-inflammatory drug known for centuries to relieve primarily muscle pain scientifically validated, inter alia, by the *Memorial Sloan Kettering Cancer Center* in New York.

- **Boswellia** (Botanical name: Boswellia serrata)

a tree growing in high altitudes of India (also Northern Africa and the Middle East), is the source of *frankincense (*we learn about in the Holy Bible) and became an important part of Indian *Ayurvedic* medicine. It has proven helpful as a very potent pain and inflammation reliever validated, inter alia, by the *University of New York* Langone Medical Center and the *Memorial Sloan Kettering Cancer Center* in New York.

Recommended **dosage** 500 mg 2-3 times daily.

- **Bromelain**

as a mixture of enzymes of pineapples have earned scientific appreciation for relieving pain, swelling, and inflammation after (cancer) surgery. Additionally, it has the reputation of detoxifying the bloodstream.

Scientifically validated, inter alia, by the *University of Maryland* Medical Center.

Recommended **dosage** 80 mg 1-2 times daily.

Bark and root of

- **Catuaba** (Botanical name: Erythroxylum catuaba)

a small tree of the Brazilian Amazonas of which bark and roots are used for pain relief in Brazil and the United States.

Scientifically validated at, inter alia, the University of Mississippi and the *Universidade do Vale do Itajai* in the Brazilian Amazon.

Recommended **dosage** 500 mg 2 times daily.

- **Chuchuhuasi** (Botanical name: Maytenus krukovii)

is probably one of the most effective natural alternatives for relieving different kinds of pain. It is especially used in Columbia, Ecuador, and above all Peru. (In fact, the name *Chuchuhuasi* is Peruvian.)

Usually the bark of this high canopy tree is used, sometimes also leaves and root. Scientifically validated, even far away at the *Tokyo College of Pharmacy* in Japan.

Recommended **dosage** decoction 1 cup/ ½ Tsp. 2-3 times daily.

- **Devil's Claw** (Botanical name: Harpagophytum procumbens)

from South Africa, has also the reputation of relieving pain. Scientifically validated, inter alia, by the *University of Maryland* Medical Center. Recommended **dosage** 300 mg 2 times daily.

- **Suma** (Botanical name: Pfaffia paniculata)

The roots of this shrubby vine, which is also called 'Brazilian Ginseng', are used for pain especially in Brazil and Peru.

In our Western hemisphere this is scientifically validated at, inter alia, the *Jefferson Medical College* in Philadelphia, PA.

Recommended **dosage** decoction 1 cup/ ½ Tsp. 2-3 times daily.

- **Tayuya** (Botanical name: Cayaponia tayuya)

a woody vine of which the roots have been used historically already for long time for pain relief not only in the Amazon region but also in the U.S.

Scientifically validated, inter alia, at the *University of Oxford* in the UK.

For recommended daily **dosage** 1g-2g 1-2 daily.

Scientifically validated by Memorial *Sloan Kettering Cancer Center,*

- **White Willow Bark** (Botanical name: Salix spp.)

is probably the best known herb for pain (and inflammation) with quite some history:

After White Willow Bark has been used for pain relief by man for millions of years (!) effectively, pharma company *Bayer* synthesized it, surrounded it with a synthetic-chemical formula, and patented it in the year of 1900 to sell it up to date as *ASPIRIN* - with all its chemical side effects. Since then, year 1900, mainstream medicine was born.

But please make no mistake: pure and natural White Willow Bark is still on the market, in the shadow of Aspirin and related chemical drugs.

For recommended daily **dosage** see label.

Scientifically validated at, inter alia, the *University of Mississippi* and the *Universidade de Vale do Itajal* in the Amazon.

- **Cat's Claw** (Botanical name: Uncuria guianensis)

from South America belongs also to this herbal wealth for pain, and inflammation. Scientifically validated at the *Memorial Sloan Kettering Cancer Center* in New York.

Recommended daily **dosage** 1000 mg up to 3 times daily.

You may also consider adding following herbs, which are not specifically known for pain relief but still helpful for this health problem:

- **_Ginger_** (Botanical name: Zingiber officinalis)

the 'root' of a plant by the botanical name of Zingiber officinalis, reduces pain, as well as inflammation and nausea scientifically validated, inter alia, by the _University of Maryland_ Medical Center.

Recommended **_dosage_** 500 mg twice daily.

When it comes to relieve **_neuropathic_** pain,

- **_Ginkgo_** (Botanical name: Ginkgo biloba)

is a scientifically validated option, according to, inter alia, _The Catholic University_ of Seoul, South Korea, and Memorial _Sloan Kettering Cancer Center_ in New York.

Recommended **_dosage_** up to 120 mg daily.

Another herb of high potency is

- **_Turmeric_** (Botanical name: Curcuma longa)

a relative of _ginger_ which gives _curry_ the flavor and yellow color, Turmeric was used since thousands of years in Indian _Ayurvedic_ medicine as well as _Traditional Chinese Medicine_ (TCM) for, inter alia, pain relief, inflammation, and digestive problems.

Scientifically validated nowadays, inter alia, at the _University of Maryland_ Medical Center.

Also, renowned _Memorial Sloan Kettering Cancer Center_ in New York has validated scientifically Turmeric being more effective and safer for pain relief than Aspirin.

In our modern times, Turmeric has also found appreciation for preventing and treating certain types of cancer (breast, skin, colon, etc.).

Recommended daily **_dosage_** 800 mg.

- ***Tart Cherries***

are another phytochemical to reduce pain with special reference to chronic inflammation, according to *Oregon Health & Science University,* the *Baylor Research Institute* in Dallas, TX, and the *University of Pennsylvania.*

Recommended daily **dosage** up to 3 times 250 mg each.

One other powerful anti-pain (and anti-inflammation) plants is

- ***Acai***

as scientifically validated at, inter alia, the *University of Arkansas* and the *Shanghai Institute of Pharmaceutical Industry.*
Also consider

- ***Vitamin D***

because a deficiency of this vitamin may lead to pain, especially of muscles and bones. According to research at, inter alia, the *University of Minnesota* Medical School.

Therefore, if your vitamin D level is too low, it is strongly recommended to balance with vitamin D containing food such as, inter alia, fatty fish and fish-liver oils, egg yolk, mushrooms, and liver. Additionally, get natural sun exposure, or take a vitamin D supplement up to 2000 I.U. (Check you Vitamin D level regularly by blood count, as it should have no less but 30 mg/ml.)

Also,

- ***Integrative Medicine***

modalities such as

- *Guided Imagery*
- *Acupuncture*
- *Massage*
- *Relaxation Response Intervention*
- *Stress Management*

are worth a try in order to help in view of additional cancer related pain relief. For details please check with the *Penny George Institute for Health and Healing* with different locations in Minnesota, specializing in these integrative medical modalities. (See also chapter *Anxiety* in this book.)

Since our body is a systemic phenomenon and therefore, any health problem should be seen from a systemic point of view, we should also understand that, according to the *Norwegian Institute of Public Health* in Bergen, Norway, there is a synergistic effect between **sleep** problems and chronic pain. I.e. poor sleep is increasing pain sensitivity – and vice-versa. This implies that in case of chronic pain, good night sleep is a most important issue.

Also, when it comes to relieving pain and anxiety after surgery, you may listen to

- ● *Music*

according to research at *Brunel University* in the UK. In fact, the researchers recommend this music therapy not only for the time *after* surgery but also before and during surgery. However, since most hospitals don't follow this advice, although scientifically validated, you the patient may only have the chance to materialize it on your own *before* and *after* surgery.

Finally, and often overlooked, is the fact that

- ● *Healthy Diet*

can lower pain sensitivity, according to research at *Ohio State University*.

As an exotic modality but, according to the *University of Kentucky Markey Cancer Center* helpful, is the

- ● *Touch Therapy 'Shin Jyutsu'*

to relieve cancer treatment side effects, especially pain and nausea.

Also, *detoxification* of the body and *anti-inflammatory* measures may relief pain.

>>><<<

See also chapters
TOXIFICATION, INFLAMMATION

SEXUAL DYSFUNCTION

There are many different ways to develop sexual dysfunction in both, men and women – physically and even more, emotionally related. More than 40% women are affected (*female sexual dystrophy*) according to *the University of Colorado, Loma Linda University* in Loma Linda, *CA,* and *Columbia University* in New York. And more than 30% of men (*erectile dysfunction*) are affected, according to the U.S. Institutes of Health.

One of the major potential causes of developing sexual dysfunction is conventional gynecological cancer treatment, including surgery, chemotherapy, and radiation. There are almost 90,000 diagnoses annually, primarily in younger and premenopausal women – especially cancer of the ovaries, uterus, vulva, vagina, and cervix.

According to research at the *University of Colorado Cancer Center* and scientific validation at *Columbia University* in New York, *Loma Linda University* in California, and the *Denver Health Medical Center* in Colorado.

In terms of natural remedies to help in these cases,

- ● **Fenugreek** (Botanical name: Trigonella foenum-graecum)

has been scientifically validated by the Australian *Universities of Sydney, Queensland,* and *Southern Queensland* to counterbalance sexual dystrophy in women. Scientifically validated at the *Memorial Sloan Kettering Cancer Center* in New York.

Recommended daily **dosage** up to 2000 mg in 3 installments.

Additionally, following libido increasing Rainforest herbs may have a positive effect on sexual dystrophy for both, men and women.

- ● **Muira puama** (Botanical name: Ptychopetalum olacoides)

also called "potency wood", promotes sexual function – according to research at the *University of Washington* in Seattle, WA and (with special reference to erectile dysfunction) also at the *Morgagni-Pierantoni Hospital* in Forli, Italy.

Recommended **dosage**: gently simmer 1 teaspoon of bark in one cup of water for 15 minutes and take 1/2 to 1 cup daily.

Another promising herb from the South American Rainforest for improving sexual performance is

- **Maca** (Botanical name: Lepidium meyenii)

according to the *Shin Medical & Aesthetic Clinic* in Torrance, CA.

Recommended **dosage**: 5-20 g daily. Stir 2 tsp of dried root powder into juice or water.

Additionally, you may also consider following modalities, according to *Mayo Clinic:*

- **Acupuncture**

especially in cases of sexual *pain* disorders.

Another modality may be

- **Yoga**

as certain subsets of yoga can channel the body's sexual energy.

Also

- **Relaxation**

as a matter of

- **Stress Release**

may help, as well as regular aerobic

- **Physical Exercise**

SKIN DAMAGES

Surgery, chemotherapy and radiation, which are the most common conventional treatment options, in many cases, may produce unsightly streaking, acne, and bruising.

Especially chemotherapy drugs attack rapidly dividing cells – not only cancer cells, but any rapidly dividing such as, inter alia, cells of the mouth lining (leading to *mouth sores),* lining of the intestines (promoting *nausea* and *vomiting) –* and also skin cells.

Radiation in fact has a devastating impact on the respective skin areas in 3 stages. First stage is that the skin becomes red and itches. Second stage may be dryness with flaking and peeling. Stage no. 3 may be scarring. In this respect, radiation can cause damages in and outside of the body which, to be sure, can also be long-term.

For damages outside, especially skin inflammation in cases of breast cancer, the *Center for Integrative Botanical Studies* in Boulder, CO, recommends topically the herb

- *Calendula* (Botanical name: Calendula officinalis)

scientifically validated at *Memorial Sloan Kettering Cancer Center* in New York.

From the same source we learn that

- *Green Tea* (Botanical name: Camellia sinensis)

may support skin from within, based on its *catechin* compound, and slow the progress of existing skin cancer by application outside. Scientifically validated at the *University of Manchester*, UK, and the *Memorial Sloan Kettering Cancer Center* in New York.

According to scientific validation by the *National Cancer Institute of the United States* and the *National Cancer Institute of Canada,*

- *Vitamin K-1*

is an excellent option to overcome these side effects naturally, by supporting the inherent healing power of the skin.

Recommended **dosage** 1000 mcg (1 g) daily, along with

- **Vitamin D**

which supports skin regeneration, preferably from sun exposure, or at least 2000 IU as a supplement.

Complemented by the European herb

- **Arnica** (Botanical name: Arnica montana)

from the herbal sunflower family because of its anti-inflammatory and anti-itching power.

For recommended daily **dosage** see label.

As well as dietary

- **Oats**

because of their moisturizing ability clearing away also dead skin cells, speeds regeneration.

Another powerful skin repair mechanism comes from Southern France – the maritime pine bark

- **Pycnogenol** (Botanical name: Pinus pinaster)

which, inter alia, supports elasticity and hydration of the skin, enhances blood flow to the skin, and protects skin against radiation.

Based on research at, inter alia, the *Leibniz Research Institute for Environmental Medicine* in Dusseldorf, Germany.

For daily **dosage** see label.

Another 'revolutionary' nutrient is

- **Procaine HCI**

composed as a blend of certain molecules and B vitamins, developed by French scientists and refined by Romanian doctor Ana Aslan for, inter alia, mood lifting, cell detoxification, is also a strong power for mental focus, and memory enhancement.

For daily **dosage** see label.

Also you may consider

- **Ultrasound**

is a very innovative mechanism for stimulating the healing process of the skin. According to research at the *University of Sheffield* and the *University of Bristo,* both UK.

SLEEP DEPRIVATION

According to the *National Sleep Foundation* in the U.S., more than half of adults have sleep problems *(insomnia)*, i.e. lacking the ability to fall, or to stay asleep. Although in fact a **symptom**, not a disorder in strict sense, it has reached *epidemic* proportions. With partly dramatic consequences for our health according to research at, inter alia, the *University of Copenhagen*, Denmark.

Sleep duration and quality of sleep can also have an impact on cancer survival, according to the *Fred Hutchinson Cancer Research Center* in Seattle, WA. It also can lower pain tolerance – based on findings of the *Norwegian Institute of Public Health* in Bergen, Norway.

Vice-versa, poor quality of sleep may support the development of colon cancer, according to research at the *Case Western Reserve University* in Cleveland, OH, and breast cancer according to *Dartmouth University* in Hanover, NH.

Very often insomnia is also related to *depression* – according to research at, inter alia, the *Sheba Medical Center* in Ramat Gan, Israel – as well as weight gain and decreased brain function – according to research at the *University of Warwick* (ranked as one of top 10 universities in the UK).

Even worse, sleep deprivation is a risk factor for premature death, according to the *University of Warwick*, and is running down our immunity, according to *Tufts University* research.

Since the quality and duration of sleep is also a matter of personal **stress** – according to the *Sleep Disorders & Research Center* at *Henry Ford Hospital* in Detroit, MI – please read the chapter on **stress** in this guide carefully.

Despite of that medical relevance, this phenomenon is poorly understood by the medical profession, as research at *Dartmouth Medical School* in Lebanon, NH, demonstrates. This is specifically problematic with respect to **cancer**.

To be sure, conventional cancer treatment may well cause sleep deprivation (insomnia). However, to overcome this side effect you better refrain from prescription sleeping pills, as taking chemical sleeping pills on a regular basis are not only addictive, they don't resolve the underlying problem.

These sleeping pills – yes – can even cause cancer – according to comprehensive research at the *Scripps Clinic Sleep Center* in San Diego, CA. Scientifically validated at renowned *Stanford University*'s Stanford Sleep Disorders Clinic.

To evade this vicious cycle of prescription sleeping pills, almost 2 million Americans choose complementary and alternative medicine for insomnia, according to the U.S. *National Center for Health Statistics* of the *Centers for Disease Control and Prevention.*

From the herbal kingdom, probably the best natural choice for a sound sleep is

- ● *Valerian* (Botanical name: Valeriana officinalis)

according to research at, inter alia, the *University of California* in Davis, CA, and *Pacific Western University* in Los Angeles, and validation by, inter alia, *Memorial Sloan Kettering Cancer Center* in New York and the *Commission E* (the European equivalent to the FDA in the U.S.).

Recommended daily *dosage* up to 1000 mg, or by drinking it as a cup of tea before bed time.

Another herb with high reputation is well known in Indian *Ayurvedic* medicine for more than 3000 years, scientifically validated at, inter alia, the *University of Michigan, Memorial Sloan Kettering Cancer Center* in New York, and *CSM Medical University* in India:

- ● *Ashwagandha* (Botanical name: Withania somnifera)

Recommended daily *dosage* of 2 times 500 mg.

Similar the results for the herb

- ● *Kava* (Botanical name: Piper methysticum)

as scientifically validated at, inter alia, *Memorial Sloan Kettering Cancer Center* in New York, and *South Dakota State University.*

Recommended daily *dosage* of 3 times daily 100 mg up to 400 mg twice daily.

However, since Kava has been questioned by FDA in late 2001/early 2002, based on potential liver problems due to Kava in Europe (without banning it in the U.S.), you may check with your healthcare provider, if this herb is right for you in your specific situation, which dosage exactly, and how long you should take it.

- **Black Cohosh** (Botanical name: Actaea racemosa)

is another herb recommended to overcome not only menopausal mood swings but also insomnia, based on research at, inter alia, the *University of Montana* in Missoula.

Recommended **dosage** of up to 40 mg twice daily.

Quite some competence in terms of natural sleep aids can also be found at *Tel Aviv University* in Israel, with respect to, inter alia, the German type of

- **Chamomile** (Botanical name: Matricaria chamomilla)

with a recommended **dosage** of either one cup of tea in the evening, or 400 mg dried herb (capsule) up to 6 times daily. Scientifically validated by, inter alia, *Memorial Sloan Kettering Cancer Center* in New York.

Also,

- **5-HTP** (Hydroxytryptophan)

a form of the amino acid of *L-Tryptophan* may help – according to research at the *Massachusetts Institute of Technology,* the *National Institutes of Health*, and *Stanford University*.

Recommended daily **dosage** up to 200 mg daily.

Equally high reputation as a sleep enhancer has

- **Melatonin**

as a hormone produced in the pineal gland during nighttime which regulates the sleep/wake cycle. If this production decreases with age (usually after 40 years), melatonin may be consumed as a supplement.

Recommended **dosage** up to 3 mg controlled-released.

Its benefit has been scientifically validated by, inter alia, by the Massachusetts *Institute of Technology, Memorial Sloan Kettering Cancer*

Center in New York and the *National Institute of Mental Health and Neurosciences* in Bangalore, India.

To get the same benefit of melatonin, you may also consider **tart cherry** juice twice a day, for potentially 2 weeks, according to research at *Louisiana State University*.

Also

- **DHA** (Docosahexaenoic Acid)

with high levels of **omega-3** supports sleep very well, according to research at the *University of Oxford* in the UK.

Recommended daily **dosage** up to 1000 mg (1 g) twice a day.

Not to forget about the so called 'anti-stress mineral'

- **Magnesium**

of which most Americans are highly deficient in their food, with approximately only half of the recommended **dosage** of 500 mg by the Magnesium Research Center at Kumamoto *University* in Japan.

Similar the situation with your

- **Copper**

level in your blood. Of which most Americans are deficient, thus being responsible for, inter alia, poor sleep. To balance it, the recommended **dosage** is 900 micrograms per day, according to research at the *University of Eastern Finland*.

Scientifically validated by the *Linus Pauling Institute* at *Oregon State University*. (Please note: Dr. Linus Pauling is a 2-time Nobel Prize laureate and founder of the *Orthomolecular Medicine*.)

While most fruits and vegetables are low in copper, following foods are especially rich in copper: beef liver (more than 4,000 micrograms per 1 oz.) and oyster meat (more than 1500 micrograms per 1 oz.), and also nuts (almonds and cashew), as well as mushrooms.

Also, to relieve insomnia *University of Chicago* School of Medicine recommends

- ## *Human Growth Hormone (HGH)*

at least if you over 40 years old.

Potential **dosage** daily 3.3 mg 1-2 times.

Finally,

- ## *Physical exercise*

regularly and aerobic, is recommended by *Mayo Clinic.* Preferably in the morning, according to *Fred Hutchinson Cancer Research Center* in Seattle and *Towson University* in Maryland.

This way your brain produces *endorphins* which make you 'happy' – the natural way. (Refrain from legal and illegal drugs promising the same result!)

Additionally, you may follow some lifestyle recommendations by the *American Academy of Sleep Medicine (AASM)* like, inter alia,

- Same routine for bedtime and getting up in the morning
- No heavy meals before bed, no caffeine, but still not hungry
- No extended exercise last 6 hours before bed
- Relax before bed, no worries
- Have a relaxing atmosphere in your bedroom (dark, cool, quiet)

Rounded up by lifestyle factors designed at *Saint Louis University*, a private university in St. Louis, Missouri. Inter alia,

- No napping after 2 p.m.
- Check your medications on sleep
- Manage stress

Also, you may adjust your sleeping time between 6 and 8 hours, according to research at the *University of Pittsburgh,* to avoid high blood pressure and cholesterol, both risk factors for heart disease – besides many other physical and mental age-related ailments, according to *University of Chicago* research. These recommendations are in line with research at *New York Presbyterian Hospital* and *Weill Medical College of Cornell University* in New York.

However, 8 hours may well be the upper limit, as a study performed by the *American Cancer Society* shows, according to which the risk of dying of cancer is 15% higher with a sleeping time of 8 ½ hours or more.

On the other hand, sleeping less than 6 hours raises the risk of hypertension, according to research at the *University of Chicago*.

Also, research at *Penn State College of Medicine* in Hershey, PA, confirms that sleep deprivation raises blood pressure and, according to the *University of Chicago Medical School*, increases the risk of Type 2 **diabetes.**

Scientifically validated, inter alia, by *Yale University* in New Haven, CT, *Northwestern University* in Evanston, IL, and the *Henry Ford Hospital* in Detroit, MI.

According to research at *Columbia University* in New York, sleeping 5 hours or less and 9 hours or more may trigger diabetes.

Also, gastrointestinal problems such as ***irritable bowel syndrome*** may arise from insomnia, based on research at *Mayo Clinic College of Medicine* in Rochester, Minnesota.

Based on research at *Harvard University*

- ***Yoga***

may help you finding sound sleep. Also,

- ***Diet***

plays a role when it comes to sleep.

You should refrain from high-fat foods such as e.g. burgers, French fries, and caffeine (beware – some prescription drugs contain caffeine!). Tryptophan-rich foods such as, inter alia, nuts, seeds, dairy products, eggs, bananas, honey and yogurt are appropriate to support sleep.

Above all – for a good quality of sleep fraternize with

- ***Nature***

in terms of, e.g., parks, beaches, etc., and also sunlight and moderate temperature according to research at the *University of Illinois* and *New York University*.

STRESS

According to the *World Health Organization (WHO)*, almost half a billion (!) people suffers from stress worldwide. As reported by the *American Institute of Stress* in Yonkers, NY, more than 40% of Americans are affected by stress, with a heavy toll on their professional and personal life.

Not only this. Based on research at the *University of Western Ontario,* Canada, *stress* is strongly linked to underlying mental health problems as *anxiety* or *depression*. Scientifically validated with respect to *depression* also at *Harvard Medical School* and *McLean Hospital* in Boston, and by the *Uniformed Services University of the Health Sciences* in Bethesda, MD. This makes these illnesses, together with *mood disorders*, a predominant causes of *chronic disease,* according to the *World Health Organization (WHO).*

Similar are the findings at the *University of Florida*, where a link was found between stress and *Alzheimer's disease.*

Stress also has a heavy impact on the emotional level, according to research and scientific validation at *Claremont Graduate University* in Claremont, CA, and the *University of Alabama* in Birmingham, AL.

Physically, there is a link between stress and *heart disease* (especially in females), according to research and scientific validation at *New York-Presbyterian Hospital/Columbia University Medical Center, Columbia University College of Physicians and Surgeons, Wake Forest University* in Winston-Salem, N.C., and the *University of Iowa.*

Stress may also cause *stroke* – according to research at the *University of Gothenburg* and *Sahlgrenska University Hospital*, both Sweden.

Similar are the results of a study elaborated at *Duke University* in Durham, N.C. demonstrating a link between stress and *diabetes.*

With respect to cancer, there is a strong relationship between stress and cancer development (especially breast cancer) according to research at, inter alia, *Carnegie Mellon University* in Pittsburgh, PA, and the *University of British Columbia* in Canada.

This has been validated by *Ohio State University* with respect to potential tumor growth in cases of melanoma.

One of probably most powerful natural remedies to relieve stress, known for more than 3000 years in Indian *Ayurvedic* medicine, is

- ***Ashwagandha*** (Botanical name: Withania somnifera)

according to research at the *University of Michigan* and *CSM Medical University* in India. Scientifically validated by *Memorial Sloan Kettering Cancer Center* in New York.

Recommended daily ***dosage*** 2 times 500 mg.

As another recommended herb

- ***Roseroot/Golden Root*** (Botanical name: Rhodiola rosea)

an arctic root from originally Siberia, has great reputation to ward off stress, anxiety, and depression, according to research at the *University of Pennsylvania* and *Columbia University* in New York. It supports the body to resist stress, according to research at the *University of Massachusetts* in Amherst, MA and scientifically validated at, inter alia, *Memorial Sloan Kettering Cancer Center* in New York.

Recommended daily ***dosage*** up to 300 mg.

Also helpful, according to the *Human Cognitive Neuroscience Unit* at the *University of Northumbria* in the United Kingdom may be

- ***Lemon Balm***

with its calming effect by boosting the relaxation-inducing neurotransmitter GABA (Gammaaminobutyric Acid), and for better accuracy of attention.

Recommended daily ***dosage*** up to 1,600 mg.

When talking about nutrients for stress relieve, we should also consider one specific herb

- ***Curcumin*** (Botanical name: Curcuma longa)

the yellow pigment in the root of the Turmeric plant which is used in Indian natural medicine (*Ayurvedic* medicine) since thousands of years.

Scientifically validated, inter alia, at the *University of Colorado*, the *Swinburne University of Technology* in Melbourne, Australia, and *Selcuk University* in Turkey.

Recommended daily **dosage** 800 mg.

Additionally, the *University of California* in Los Angeles (UCLA) has done research on following 4 remedies worth to try:

- **Ginseng** (Panax ginseng)

which assists adrenal glands to produce the stress hormones adrenaline and cortisol.

Recommended daily **dosage** up to 500 mg.

Excellent reputation to relieve anxiety, depression and cognitive decline has the bark of

- **Magnolia** (Botanical name: Magnolia stellata)

This is known for some 2000 years and has been validated by, inter alia, the *Institute for Traditional Medicine* in Portland, Oregon.

Recommended **dosage** 30 mg up to 3 times daily.

Similar are the results for the herb

- **Kava** (Botanical name: Piper methysticum)

as scientifically validated at, inter alia, *Memorial Sloan Kettering Cancer Center* in New York and *South Dakota State University*.

Recommended **dosage** up to 400 mg twice daily.

However, since Kava has been questioned by FDA in late 2001/early 2002, based on potential liver problems due to Kava in Europe (without banning it in the U.S.), you may check with your healthcare provider, if this herb is right for you in your specific situation, which dosage exactly, and how long you should take it.

Similar results with a calming effect have been achieved with 4 cups of

- **_Black Tea_** (botanical name: Camellia sinensis)

according to research at the _City University London_ in the UK.

With same effect validated for

- **_Green Tea_** (botanical name: Camellia sinensis)

at the _University of Tokyo_ in Japan, as well as _Memorial Sloan Kettering Cancer Center_ in New York. Based on the amino acid L-theanine which is found exclusively in green tea and which triggers natural chemical changes in the brain.

Please note: The calming effect of black and green tea will be active after steeping for at least 5 minutes. This effect is dependent on individual metabolism.

Even

- **_Walnuts_**

may help to relieve stress, according to research at, inter alia, Pennsylvania _State University_.

Also, the hormone

- **_DHEA_** (Dehydroepiandrosterone)

plays a positive role in the process of relieving anxiety naturally – according to research at _Yale University_ and the _Veterans Affairs New England Healthcare System_ in West Haven, CT.

Recommended daily **_dosage_** 100 mg.

Equally important is

- **_Magnesium_**

also called 'anti-stress mineral' of which most Americans are highly deficient in their food, with approximately only half of the recommended **_dosage_** of up to 500 mg. Scientifically validated, inter alia, at the Magnesium Research Center of _Kumamoto University_ in Japan.

Another option is the amino acid

- ***Tyrosine***

in stress situations.

Recommended daily ***dosage*** 100 mg.

Supported by another amino acid

- ***DLPA*** (DL-phenylalamine)

which is converted into Tyrosine by the body.

Recommended daily ***dosage*** up to 1000 mg. (Prohibited in case of hypertension.)

You may also try

- ***St. John's Wort*** (Botanical name: Hypericum perforatum)

Scientifically validated at *Memorial Sloan Kettering Cancer Center* in New York.

Also used for depression, with special reference to the *Wake Forest Baptist Medical Center* in Winston-Salem, N.C.

Recommended daily ***dosage*** up to 300 mg.

Another 'revolutionary' nutrient is

- ***Procaine HCI***

Composed as a blend of certain molecules and B vitamins, it was developed by French scientists and refined by Romanian doctor Ana Aslan for, inter alia, stress, cell detoxification, is also a strong power for mental focus, memory enhancement and mood lifting.

For daily ***dosage*** see label.

According to the *Walter Reed National Military Medical Center* in Bethesda, MD, also turning to

- **Music**

may relieve stress, anxiety and depression at home or wherever you are. What kind of music? Just what you like most! When and how long? You decide.

This self-administered therapy may not only lower high blood pressure, according to the *Council for High Blood Pressure Research* of the *American Heart Association,* but is also specifically helpful to relieve anxiety and pain before, at, or after surgery, according to research at *Brunel University* in the UK.

Finally,

- **Physical Exercise**

at least 5 days a week with 45 minutes each, is eliciting a *relaxation response* which helps to overcome stress, according to, inter alia, *Harvard University,* the *University of Maryland* and *Massachusetts General Hospital.*

With additionally 2 days of strength training, 40 minutes each.

Scientifically validated, inter alia, by the *American College of Sports Medicine*, largest sports medicine and exercise science organization worldwide.

>>><<<

See also chapters
ANXIETY, DEPRESSION, MOOD SWINGS

TOXICATION

Those chemical drugs used for chemotherapy belong to the most toxic ones modern medicine has ever developed, to get cancer patients on *remission*. Same situation is with radiation (radiology), as far as toxic consequences for body and mind is concerned.

If you try to counterbalance this effect with other chemical medication, you are in a vicious cycle. Your only way out are natural modalities like, e.g.

- ● ***Bromelain***

a pineapple enzyme, according to research at the *University of Maryland* Medical Center and scientifically validated at *Memorial Sloan Kettering Cancer Center* in New York.

Recommended daily ***dosage*** up to 500 mg.

The *University of Maryland* has also validated

- ● ***Dandelion root*** (Botanical name: Taraxacum officinale)

a member of the herbal sunflower family and known as a folk remedy in Europe since 15th century for – not only but also – detoxification of the liver and kidneys, etc. and therefore, specifically predestined for drug-related detoxification.

Recommended daily ***dosage*** up to 500 mg.

An equally powerful detoxifier is the ancient Greek and Egyptian herb is

- ● ***Aloe vera*** (Botanical name: Aloe arborescens & Aloe barbadensis)

In fact, it is one of the best herbs for all ages and through all bodily detoxification channels as the liver, the lymph system, the skin and the bowels.

Additionally to its virtues of being anti-inflammatory and supportive in terms of skin renewal, digestion, and immunity. Comprehensively researched at, inter alia, *Tufts University*.

Recommended daily ***dosage*** up to 5000 mg.

From India is the very potent historic herb

- **Ashwagandha** (Botanical name: Withania somnifera)

used in Ayurvedic *medicine* since 2000 years, known also by the name 'Indian ginseng' and 'Indian Winter Cherry' which helps for detoxification, chemotherapy and radiation included.

Recommended daily **dosage** up to 500 mg 2 times daily.

Finally, see a sample of historically evidenced-based Rainforest herbs which help for detoxification, with special reference to liver cleansing. In alphabetical order:

- **Artichoke** (Botanical name: Cynara scolymus)
- **Amor Seco** (Botanical name: Desmodium adscendens)
- **Bitter Melon** (Botanical name: Momoridica charantia)
- **Cat's Claw** (Botanical name: Uncaria tomentosa)
- **Chanca Piedra** (Botanical name: Phyllantus niruri)
- **Fedegoso** (Botanical name: Cassia occidentalis)
- **Nettle** (Botanical name: Urtica dioica)
- **Samambaia** (Botanical name: Polypodium decumanum)
- **Sarsaparilla** (Botanical name: Smilax officinalis)
- **Tayuya** (Cayaponia tayuya)

Another natural substance to detoxify your body has been thoroughly researched at *George Washington University* and the *University of Albany*:

- **Vitamin B-3** (Niacin)

to flush toxins from different fat tissues and other fatty organs as, e.g., brain.

Recommended daily **dosage** 500-1000 mg.

It was, inter alia, 2 times Nobel Prize laureate from *Oregon State University* and founder of the *Orthomolecular Medicine*, Dr. Linus Pauling, who favored

- ***Vitamin C***

as one of the best detoxification remedies (and cancer fighter) nature has given us. Dr. Pauling recommended a daily ***dosage*** of (intravenous) 10,000 mg (10 g).

In a large chemo preventive study in Europe (EUROSCAN) the amino acid variants both,

- ***N-Acetylcysteine*** (NAC)

(recommended daily **dosage** up to 600 mg) as an amino acid precursor to

- ***Glutathione***

(recommended daily ***dosage*** up to 500 mg)

Both have been successfully tested for detoxification.

Based on research at, inter alia, the *University of Maryland* and scientifically validated at *Memorial Sloan Kettering Cancer Center,* the U.S. *National Cancer Institute* and *Mayo Clinic, etc.*

The antioxidant activity of Glutathione is specifically increased by

- ***Milk Thistle*** (Botanical name: Silynum marianum)

the no. 1 herb for detoxification for the body (liver, kidneys, colon, etc.) used since 2000 years.

Recommended daily ***dosage*** up to 1000 mg.

Also,

- ***Green Tea*** (Botanical name: Camellia sinensis)

has been researched at, inter alia, the *University of Arizona* Cancer Center, and scientifically validated at *Memorial Sloan Kettering Cancer Center* in New York to support the production of enzymes used by the body for

detoxification, and fight against cancer cells because of the substance *catechins* prevalent in green tea. That's why cancer cases in Japan and China are lower than the western industrialized world.
Scientifically validated by the U.S. *National Cancer Institute* and the *American Association for Cancer Research (AACR) in Philadelphia, PA*. Another powerful detox agent according to, inter alia, the *National University of Ireland*, and is the freshwater algae

- **Chlorella**

which contains high concentrations of Vitamin C and Vitamin B-complex, both important detox agents.

Recommended daily **dosage** up to 3 x 1000 mg.

Another important, and well researched, herb for detoxification is

- **Curcumin** (Botanical name: Curcuma longa)

according to research at, inter alia, the *University of Maryland*, which promotes the production of bile in the gallbladder, and which gives

- **Turmeric** (Botanical name: Curcuma longa)

used in India for medicinal purposes in *Ayurvedic* medicine since millennia, its yellow color.

Recommended **dosage** up to 800 mg each/alternative.

Well researched at, inter alia, King *George's Medical University* and the *International Institute of Herbal Medicine*, both in the city of Lucknow, India. And scientifically validated at *Memorial Sloan Kettering Cancer Center*.

- **Omega-3**

fatty acids have also been validated as a detox agent based on research at, inter alia, *Oregon State University*.

Recommended daily **dosage** up to 1000 mg.

Lots of

- *Spring Water*

and *organic*

- *Fruit/Vegetables*

in your diet, also in form of *juice*, are highly recommended. Not only for the antioxidants contained but also for their content of

- *Fiber*

as a detoxifying agent, according to *Mayo Clinic*. Here are just some of the high fiber fruits and vegetables:

- Sesame seeds
- Nuts, such as
    - Almonds
    - Pistachios
    - Walnuts
    - Peanuts
    - Cashews
- Green peas
- Garlic
- Okra
- Rye bread
- Soybeans
- Avocados
- Celery seeds
- Lemons
- Raisins

The value of

- *Asparagus* (Botanical name: Asparagus officinalis)

Is given not only as an antioxidant to support our biological system and as a 'super food' to challenge chronic disease, including – colon-, heart-, prostate-, breast-, lung-, and other cancers. It is also as an excellent aid for detoxification. According to research at, inter alia, the *University of California* in Los Angeles *(UCLA)*.

Additionally, you may eat at least once per week

- ### *Cruciferous Vegetables*

such as broccoli, kale, cabbage, cauliflower, Brussels sprouts – also called the 'cabbage family' – , which are very supportive for the whole biological system of your body and for detoxification. Based on comprehensive research over a time of more than 20 years at *Johns Hopkins University* in Baltimore, MD. Scientifically validated also by, inter alia, the *Dana-Farber Cancer Institute* in Boston, MA.

Another 'revolutionary' nutrient is

- ### *Procaine HCI*

Composed as a blend of certain molecules and B vitamins, it was developed by French scientists and refined by Romanian doctor Ana Aslan for, inter alia, cell detoxification, is also a strong power for mental focus, memory enhancement and mood lifting.

For daily *dosage* see label.

WEIGHT GAIN

According to the U.S. *Centers for Disease Control and Prevention (CDC)*, 35% of U.S. adults – i.e. some 80 millions – are *obese*. (Obesity means 30% more weight than normal.) There are $150 billion annual medical costs involved.

Being obese is not only a risk factor for cardiovascular disease as validated by research at, inter alia, *University College London*, UK. According to, inter alia, the *American Cancer Society* and *Cancer Research UK,* it may also increase the risk of cancer severely.

This is in line with the scientific findings at *Fred Hutchinson Cancer Research Center* in Seattle, WA, that overweight/obese menopausal women are at increased risk of developing breast cancer.

Even worse, based on research of the *London School of Hygiene & Tropical Medicine* in the UK, there is a potential risk increase of 133% for esophageal cancer, 131% for endometrial (uterus) cancer, 100% gallbladder cancer.

Also, latest findings at the *University of Regensburg* in Germany came to the conclusion that being overweight/obese can lead to certain types of brain tumor.

In a nutshell, according to the *International Agency for Research on Cancer*, almost 500,000 new cancer cases per year are attributable to overweight/obesity. This is a total of 3.6% of all cancer cases globally. In North America alone, more than 100,000 obesity-related cancer cases strike.

However, it is not only the risk of new cancer cases related to increased weight/obesity; it is also the *recurrence* of, e.g. breast cancer, related to research at *Harvard University* in cooperation with renowned *Dana-Farber Cancer Center* in Boston, MA.

Not enough: according to a meta analysis of the *National Center for Health Statistics* and the *Centers for Disease Control and Prevention* in Atlanta, GA, the link between obesity and premature death has been scientifically validated.

Still, obesity is one of the leading *preventable* health problems. Most doctors do not advise their patients how to get rid of overweight.

This is especially problematic in those cases where chemotherapy is applied. Although chemotherapy in some cases is leading to weight loss, it is primarily the cause for weight gain. According to research at *Thomas Jefferson University* in Philadelphia, PA, chemotherapy can lead to a weight gain of 10 pounds in first year of treatment.

However, under no condition should you swallow anti-obesity drugs because of dramatic side effects. That's why, according to the *European Medicines Agency* (the European pendent to the U.S. FDA), these drugs are banned in Europe.

On the other hand, just focusing on low-fat diet alone is not a conclusive answer, according to research at *Harvard University* and *Brigham & Women's Hospital.*

Unfortunately, there is no 'magic bullet' solution for reducing weight; rather, a more comprehensive approach is needed in terms of remedies and modalities. As pointed out at the 2015 *Plymouth Obesity, Diabetes and Metabolic Syndrome Symposium* by, inter alia, *Plymouth University, Peninsula Collegel of Medicine and Dentistry, University of Liverpool, King's College Hospital, Institute of Cardiovascular Medical Sciences Glasgow.*

Doing justice, according to the *University of Queensland*, Australia, an appropriate level of

- *Vitamin B*

especially folic acid (vitamin B-9) and vitamin B-12 can decrease weight gain and your body mass index (BMI), which is of special relevance in North America where a too high BMI causes some 500,000 new cancer cases (with more women than men).

Supplement with vitamin-B-complex. For appropriate ***dosage*** see label.

- *Vitamin D*

is equally important for weight control, according to research at the *University of Missouri.*

Recommended daily ***dosage*** 2000 IU or moderate exposure to sunshine.

Most important, and at the same time most deficient vitamin in obese people is

- **Vitamin E**

This deficiency is responsible for ailments summarized as *metabolic syndrome,* including cancer, heart disease and diabetes. According to research at, inter alia, the Linus Pauling Institute at *Oregon State University* in Corvallis, OR.

Recommended daily **dosage** up to 1000 IU.

Another important substance for your weight control according to, inter alia, *Tulane University* and the *University of Massachusetts* research, is

- **Fiber**

Why? If your weight goes up or down, is primarily dependent on the activity of the trillions of gut bacteria in your body which are responsible for stimulating or preventing food from breaking down.

Foods with high levels of soluble fiber like nuts, seeds, oat bran, barley, lentils, beans, carrots, blueberries and apples are restricting weight gain by improving gut health, based on research at *Georgia State University.* Scientifically validated, inter alia, by research at *Washington University* in St. Louis.

In this respect, fiber is a kind of 'catalyst' in a positive way.

Unlike manifold popular belief, Irish

- **Potato**

extract helps reducing body weight, according to *McGill University* research.

Same is with

- **Green Leafy Vegetables**

such as spinach, lettuce, etc. to keep down weight, according to meta-analysis at, inter alia, the *University of Cambridge* and the *University of Southampton,* both in the UK. Validated, as far as spinach is concerned, by research at *Louisiana State University* and the *University of Lund* in Sweden.

And yes, an

- ● **Apple**

a day can also help to keep obesity at bay.

Especially *Granny Smith*, according to research at *Washington State University*.

Same is with

- ● **Blueberries**

according to research at *Texas Woman's University* in Denton, TX,

Also dried

- ● **Prunes**

are good for weight decrease, according to research at the *University of Liverpool*, UK, by curbing appetite the natural way.

- ● **Green Tea** (Botanical name: Camellia sinensis)

enriched with the substance *catechin* as found in Chinese green tea, supports weight management, according to *Peking University*. Scientifically validated at *Memorial Sloan Kettering Cancer Center* in New York.

- ● **Nuts**

such as cashews, Brazil nuts, almonds, pecans, walnuts, pistachios, etc. are another dietary support to manage weight, according to *Loma Linda University* in California.

- ● **Capsaicin**

derived from the fruit *capsicum* (chili peppers) helps to manage weight, according to findings at the *University of Wyoming*, USA, the *University of Vienna* in Austria, and *Manchester Metropolitan University* in the UK.

Scientifically validated at *Memorial Sloan Kettering Cancer Center* in New York.

Capsaicin, the molecule in chili peppers, may prevent overeating – at least, according to a most recent study elaborated by the *University of Adelaide* and the *South Australian Health and Medical Research Institute,* both in Adelaide, Australia, and funded by the *Royal Adelaide Hospital.*

Basically, fruits and vegetables are the best nutrition for weight loss, with still saving all essential nutrients our body needs for its biochemical existence. Although, according to research at *E-Da Hospital* in Taiwan, being vegetarian or vegan (latter with no animal food at all) leads to the best results, this may not be considered mandatory.

Established for thousands of years in evidence-based *Traditional Chinese Medicine* (TCM), the herb

- **Thunder God Vine** (Botanical name: *Tripterygium wilfordii)*

can cut obesity almost in half because of its compound *celastrol* by enhancing the appetite-suppressing hormone *leptin* – according to research at *Boston Children's Hospital* and *Harvard Medical School,*

For recommended daily **dosage** see label.

In terms of weight-controlling fruits and vegetables

- **Grapefruit**

supports fat reduction, according to recent research at the *University of California in Berkeley.*

True, according to research at, inter alia, the *E-Da Hospital* in Taiwan, a

- **Vegan Diet**

(a diet without any animal-based food but only fruits and d vegetables) achieves the most weight loss. In addition, endometrial cancer can be warded off according to, inter alia, research at the *IRCCS-Instituto de*

Ricerche Farmacologiche Mario Negri inMilan, Italy. However, vegans are lacking essential nutrients like, e.g. vitamin B-12 your body cannot exist on.

On the other hand,

- *Mediterranean Diet*

a diet with lots of fruits, vegetables, whole grains, nuts, grains, and olive oil serves the same purpose and provides all nutrients the body needs – as scientifically validated by, inter alia, *Harvard University.*

Also, according to a most recent study from the *University of Birmingham* in the UK and scientifically validated by *Mayo Clinic*, 500 ml (17 fl oz) of spring

- *Water*

before each meal may support weight loss.

In this context, it may still be appreciated that, according to research at the *Canadian Hospital for Sick Children Research Institute* in Toronto, and *McMaster University* in Hamilton, Ontario, commercial diet programs with sophistically sounding brand names are not an alternative to real natural nutrients, as recommended in this book.

And for the night, research at *Aarhus University* in Denmark recommends 1-3 mg of

- *Melatonin*

to lose weight during sleep. Scientifically validated at *Memorial Sloan Kettering Cancer Center* in New York.

These diet recommendations shall be rounded up by appropriate

- *Physical Exercise*

But which exercise is 'appropriate' – strength, endurance, or a mixture of both?

According to the first clinical study of this kind, elaborated at the *University of Madrid* and *La Paz University Hospital* in Spain, and validated by the *American Physiological Society (APS)* and the *University College London in* the UK, any kind of physical exercise with less sitting in leisure time – along with a healthy diet – supports weight loss. Validated inter alia by the *University of Pittsburgh* School of Medicine.

Based on research of *Stanford University* School of Medicine, more than half of American women do not exercise in their leisure time at all.

According to same research, lack of exercise is even more problematic than over-eating, when it comes to overweight/obesity.

The *American Cancer Society* recommends at least 150 minutes of moderate, or 75 minutes of vigorous physical activity per week for adults, for children and teens at least 1 hour moderate 4 days, and vigorous 3 days per week.

However, when talking about 'healthy diet', it is a myth to believe *diet* soda should be part of that. Dead wrong. According to research at, inter alia, the *University of Texas* Health Science Center in San Antonio, TX, diet soda is counterproductive by, yes, expanding waistlines.

Same is with poor sleep, leading to weight gain according to, inter alia, the *National Autonomous University of Mexico*. Vice-versa, to control weight, a sound sleep pattern is inevitable, according to the *American College of Physicians*. (See also chapter *Sleep Deprivation*.)

Weight gain is also associated with *osteoporosis* (see chapter *Osteoporosis*.)

Moderate

- ***Sun Exposure***

is no less important, according to research at *Telethon Kids Institute* in Perth, Australia, when it comes to fight weight gain.

Because moderate sun exposure of any part of the body releases a natural compound named *nitric oxide, which* reduces weight.

If you follow these recommendations above in case of a weight problem, this will also improve your *mood*, and your *sleep*, according to research at the Perelman School of Medicine at the *University of Pennsylvania*. (See chapters *Mood Swings* and *Sleep Deprivation* in this book.)

In a nutshell, while all of the above mentioned remedies and modalities may well be worth to be considered, a balanced *diet* and *exercise* are the profound pillars to control healthy weight.

>>><<<

For WEIGHT LOSS see chapter CACHEXIA

REFERENCES

In most scientific books, references are stated in form of (peer-reviewed) articles.

However, in these cases, the respective researcher/s may have already come to new conclusions – published in his next paper you have no access to.

Not only this, the researcher/s are an integrative part of a comprehensive medical unity with colleagues who may contributed to the findings in one or another way as well, even if they are not mentioned as 'et al.'

Therefore, it is much more helpful to learn about the research behind in its whole complexity of the respective medical school or other research body – with the chance to contact them and tap their research status up-to-the-minute.

For this purpose, all medical schools and other research institutions referred to in this guide are listed comprehensively with their location in the following.

U.S. & INTERNATIONAL
MEDICAL SCHOOLS & RESEARCH INSTITUTIONS
referred to in this book
(In alphabetical order)

➔ For all universities and colleges named as reference in this guide the respective department is *Medical School/School of Medicine/College of Medicine,* etc. which, therefore, has not been articulated specifically. I.e., when following up these references, please check with the respective medical department of the universities or colleges you want to communicate.

➔ To preserve scientific independence, only renowned universities and research institutions globally have been accepted by the author. No industries or other commercial bodies, etc.

U.S.A.

- American Association for the Study of Liver Diseases, Alexandria, VA
- American Academy of Sleep Medicine, Darien, IL
- American Association for Cancer Research, Philadelphia, PA
- American Association for the Study of Liver Diseases, Alexandria, VA
- American Cancer Society, Bradenton, FL
- American College of Gastroenterology, Las Vegas, NV
- American College of Physicians, Philadelphia, PA
- American College of Sports Medicine, Indianapolis, IN
- American Council on Exercise, San Diego, CA
- American Heart Association, Dallas, TX
- American Herbalist Guild, Halifax, VA
- American Holistic Center Chicago, Chicago, IL
- American Institute of Stress, Yonkers, NY
- American Physical Therapy Association, Alexandria, VA
- American Physiological Society, Bethesda, MD
- American Psychological Association, Washington, D.C.
- American Psychosomatic Society, McLean, VA
- Appalachian State University, Boone, NC
- Arizona State University, Tempe, AZ
- Association of Jesuit Colleges and Universities, Washington, D.C.
- Association of Reproductive Health Professionals, Washington, D.C.
- Auburn University, Auburn, AL
- Baptist Cardiac and Vascular Institute, Miami, FL
- Baylor Research Institute, Dallas, TX
- Beth Israel Deaconess Medical Center, Boston, MA
- Boston Children's Hospital, Boston, MA
- Boston University, Boston, MA
- Boston VA Hospital, Boston, MA
- Brigham & Women's Hospital, Boston, MA
- Brigham Young University Hawaii, Laie, HI
- Brown University, Providence, RI
- California State University, Long Beach, CA
- Cancer Prevention Institute of California, Fremont, CA
- Cardiac and Vascular Institute, Miami, FL
- Carnegie Mellon University, Pittsburgh, PA
- Case Western Reserve University, Cleveland, OH
- Center for Effective CFS/Fibromyalgia Therapies, Annapolis, MD
- Center for Integrative Botanical Studies, Boulder, CO

- Center for Mind-Body Medicine, Washington, D.C.
- Center for Natural Medicine, Portland, OR
- Center for Science in the Public Interest, Washington, D.C.
- Centers for Disease Control and Prevention (CDC), Atlanta, GA
- Children's Hospital and Research Center Oakland, Oakland, CA
- Claremont Graduate University, Claremont, CA
- Cleveland Clinic, Cleveland, OH
- Columbia University, New York City, NY
- Cooper Aerobics Center, Dallas, TX
- Cornell University, Ithaca, NY
- Creighton University, Omaha, NE
- Dana-Farber Cancer Institute, Boston, MA
- Denver Health Medical Center, Denver, CO
- Dartmouth Geisel School of Medicine, Lebanon, NH
- Dartmouth Institute for Health Policy and Clinical Practice, Lebanon, NH
- Dartmouth Norris Cotton Cancer Center, Manchester, NH
- Dartmouth University, Hanover, NH
- Duke University, Durham, N.C.
- Elmhurst Hospital Center, New York City, NY
- Emory University, Atlanta, GA
- Florida Atlantic University, Boca Raton, FL
- Florida State University, Tallahassee, FL
- Fox Chase Cancer Center, Philadelphia, PA
- Fred Hutchinson Cancer Research Center, Seattle, WA
- Georgetown University, Washington, D.C.
- George Washington University, Washington, D.C.
- Georgia Institute of Technology, Atlanta, GA
- Georgia Regents University, Augusta, GA
- Georgia State University, Atlanta, GA
- Glendale Memorial Medical Center, Glendale, CA
- Grand Forks Human Nutrition Research Center, Grand Forks, ND
- Harbor-UCLA Medical Center, Torrance, CA
- Harvard University, Cambridge, MA
- Helen Hayes Hospital, Haverstraw, NY
- Henry Ford Hospital, Detroit, MI
- Hospital for Special Surgery, New York City, NY
- Immune Recovery Clinic, Atlanta, GA
- Indiana University, Bloomington, IN
- Indiana University School of Public Health, Bloomington, IN
- Institute for Cancer Research, New York, NY
- Institute for Traditional Medicine, Portland, OR

- Iowa College of Medicine, Iowa City, IA
- Jefferson Medical College, Philadelphia, PA
- Jesuit University, Wheeling, WV
- Johns Hopkins University, Baltimore, MD
- Kellman Center for Progressive Medicine, New York, NY
- Loma Linda University, Loma Linda, CA
- Long Island University, New York City, NY
- Louisiana State University, Baton Rouge, LA
- Massachusetts General Hospital, Boston, MA
- Massachusetts Institute of Technology, Cambridge, MA
- Mayo Clinic, Rochester, MN
- McLean Hospital, Boston, MA
- Medical College of Georgia, Atlanta, GA
- Medical College of Virginia, Richmond, VA
- Medical College of Wisconsin, Milwaukee, WI
- Metropolitan State University, Denver, CO
- Moffitt Cancer Center, Tampa, FL
- Monell Chemical Senses Center, Philadelphia, PA
- Mountainwest Institute of Herbal Sciences, Salt Lake City, UT
- National Association for Continence, Spartanburg, SC
- National Cancer Institute (U.S. Department of Health and Human Services), Bethesda, MD
- National Center for Health Statistics, Atlanta, GA
- National Headache Foundation, Chicago, IL
- National Institute for Mental Health, Rockville, MD
- National Institute of Aging, Bethesda, MD
- National Institute of Diabetics and Digestive and Kidney Diseases (U.S. Department of Health and Human Services), Bethesda, MD
- National Institute on Drug Abuse, Bethesda, MD
- National Institutes of Health, Bethesda, MD
- National Sleep Foundation, Arlington, VA
- Nemours Foundation, Jacksonville, FL
- New England Center for Headache, Stamfort, CT
- New York Presbyterian Hospital, New York City, NY
- New York School of Career and Applied Studies, New York City, NY
- New York State Institute for Basic Research in Developmental Disabilities, Staten Island, NY
- New York University, New York City, NY
- North American Menopause Society, Mayfield Heights, OH
- Northwestern University, Evanston, IL
- Ohio State University, Columbus, OH
- Oklahoma State University, Stillwater, OK

- Oregon Health & Science University, Portland, OR
- Oregon State University, Corvallis, OR
- Pace University, New York City, NY
- Pacific Western University, Los Angeles, CA
- PATH Medical Center, New York City, NY
- Penn State College of Medicine, Hershey, PA
- Pennsylvania State University, State College, PA
- Penny George Institute for Health & Healing, Minnesota
- Presbyterian Hospital, New York City, NY
- Radiological Society of North America, Oak Brook, IL
- Rehabilitation Institute of Chicago, Chicago, IL
- Robert Wood Johnson Medical School, Brunswick, NJ
- Rockefeller University, New York City, NY
- Rush University, Chicago, IL
- Saint Louis University, St. Louis, MO
- San Francisco Veterans Affairs Medical Center, San Francisco, CA
- Scripps Clinic Sleep Center, San Diego, CA
- Scripps Research Institute, Jupiter, FL
- Shin Medical & Aesthetic Clinic, Torrance, CA
- South Dakota State University, Brookings, SD
- Stanford University, Stanford, CA
- Sutter Center for Integrative Health, Davis, CA
- Tahoma Clinic, Tukwila, WA
- Temple University, Philadelphia, PA
- Texas A&M University, College Station, TX
- Texas Woman's University, Denton, TX
- Thomas Jefferson University, Philadelphia, PA
- Touro College & University System, New York City, NY
- Trust for America's Health (TFAH), Washington, D.C.
- Tufts University, Boston, MA
- Uniformed Services University of the Health Sciences, Bethesda, MD
- University of Alabama, Birmingham, AL
- University at Albany, Albany, NY
- University of Arizona, Tucson, AZ
- University of Arkansas, Fayetteville, AK
- University of Arkansas, Little Rock, AK
- University of Bridgeport, Bridgeport, CT
- University of Buffalo, Buffalo, NY
- University of California, Berkeley, CA
- University of California, Davis, CA
- University of California, Irvine, CA
- University of California, Los Angeles, CA

- University of California, San Diego, CA
- University of California, San Francisco
- University of Chicago, Chicago, IL
- University of Cincinnati, Cincinnati, OH
- University of Colorado, Boulder, CO
- University of Fayetteville, Fayetteville, AK
- University of Houston, Houston, TX
- University of Illinois, Chicago, IL
- University of Iowa, Iowa City, IA
- University of Florida, Gainesville, FL
- University of Georgia, Athens, GA
- University of Kansas, Kansas City, KS
- University of Kentucky Markey Cancer Center, Lexington, KY
- University of Maryland, College Park, MD
- University of Massachusetts, Amherst, MA
- University of Miami, Miami, FL
- University of Michigan, Ann Arbor, MI
- University of Michigan Comprehensive Cancer Center, Ann Arbor, MI
- University of Minnesota, Minneapolis, MN
- University of Minnesota, St. Paul, MN
- University of Mississippi, Oxford, MS
- University of Missouri, Columbia, MO
- University of Montana, Missoula, MT
- University of New York, Syracuse, NY
- University of North Carolina, Chapel Hill, NC
- University of Pennsylvania, Philadelphia, PA
- University of Pittsburgh, Pittsburgh, PA
- University of Rochester, Rochester, NY
- University of South Carolina, Columbia, SC
- University of Tennessee, Knoxville, TN
- University of Texas, Austin, TX
- University of Texas, Dallas, TX
- University of Texas, Galveston, TX
- University of Texas, San Antonio, TX
- University of Utah, Salt Lake City, UT
- University of Virginia, Charlottesville, VA
- University of Washington, Seattle, WA
- University of Wisconsin, Madison, WI
- University of Wyoming, Laramie, WY
- Utah Pain Research Center, Salt Lake City, UT
- Vanderbilt University, Nashville, TN

- Veterans Affairs New England Healthcare System, West Haven, CT
- Vitamin D Council, San Luis Obispo, CA
- Wake Forest Baptist Medical Center, Winston-Salem, NC
- Wake Forest University, Winston-Salem, NC
- Walter Reed National Military Medical Center, Bethesda, MD
- Washington State University, Pullman, WA
- Washington State University, Spokane, WA
- Washington University, St. Louis, MO
- Weill Cornell Medical College, New York City, NY
- Wheeling Jesuit University, Wheeling, WV
- West Virginia University, USA
- Worcester Polytechnic Institute, Worcester, MA
- Yale University, New Haven, CT
- YMCA, Boothbay Harbor, ME

INTERNATIONAL

- Aarhus University , Aarhus, Denmark
- Aberdeen Royal Infirmary, Aberdeen UK
- Akita University, Akita, Japan
- Alexandria University, Alexandria, Egypt
- Al-Fateh University, Tripoli, Libya
- American University of Beirut, Beirut, Lebanon
- Australian Catholic University, Banyo, Australia
- Australian National University, Canberra, Australia
- Beijing Institute of Cancer Research, Beijing, China
- British Heart Foundation, Sheldon Birmingham, UK
- Brunel University, Uxbridge, UK
- Calgary University, Calgary, Canada
- Camilo Jose Cela University, Madrid, Spain
- Canadian Hospital for Sick Children Research Institute, Toronto, Canada
- Cancer Research UK, London, UK
- Catholic University, Leuven, Belgium
- Catholic University of Seoul, Seoul, South Korea
- Chieti-Pescara University, Chieti, Italy
- Chinese University of Hong Kong, Hong Kong
- City University London, London, UK
- CSM Medical University, Lucknow, India
- Daejeon University, Daejeon, South Korea
- Defence Institute of Physiology and Allied Sciences, Delhi, India
- Ebetsu University, Ebetsu, Japan

- E-Da Hospital, Kaohsiung City, Taiwan
- Erciyes University, Kayseri, Turkey
- European Medicines Agency, London, UK
- Garden Healing Clinic, Vancouver, Canada
- Glasgow Caledonian University, Glasgow, UK
- Goethe University, Frankfurt, Germany
- Griffith University, Nathan, Australia
- Harokopio University, Athens, Greece
- Hospital Dr. Joseph Trueta, Girona, Spain
- Hospital Universitario Ramon y Cajal, Madrid, Spain
- Hospital Universitario Reina Sofia de Cordoba, Cordoba, Spain
- Imperial College, London, UK
- Institut de Cancerologie de l'Ouest, Nantes, France
- Institute for Quality and Efficiency in Health Care, Cologne, Germany
- Institute of Cardiovascular Medical Sciences, Glasgow, UK
- International Agency for Research on Cancer, Lyon, France
- International Institute of Herbal Medicine, Lucknow, India
- International Osteoporosis Foundation, Nyon, Switzerland
- IRCCS-Instituto de Ricerche Farmacologiche Mario Negri, Milan, Italy
- Italian Research Institute on Food and Nutrition, Rome, Italy
- Jagiellonian University, Krakow, Poland
- Jamaia Hamdard University, Delhi, India
- Karolinska Institute, Solna, Sweden
- Keiju Medical Center, Nanao City, Japan
- Keio University, Keio, Japan
- King George's Medical University, Lucknow, India
- King's College, London, UK
- Konkuk University, Seoul, South Korea
- Kumamoto University, Kumamoto, Japan
- Kyungpook University, Buk-gu, South Korea
- La Paz University Hospital, La Paz, Spain
- Leeds Institute of Rheumatic and Muskosceletal Medicine, Leeds, UK
- Leibniz Research Institute for Environmental Medicine, Dusseldorf, Germany
- Leiden University, Leiden, Netherlands
- London Metropolitan University, London, UK
- London School of Hygiene & Tropical Medicine, London, UK
- Maastricht University, Maastricht, Netherlands
- Manchester Metropolitan University, Manchester, UK
- Marselisborg Unversity Hospital, Marselisborg, Denmark

- Max Planck Institute for Infection Biology, Berlin, Germany
- Max Planck Institute of Psychiatry, Munich, Germany
- McGill University, Montreal, Canada
- McMaster University, Hamilton, Canada
- Memorial University of Newfoundland, St. John's, Canada
- Mimasaka Women's College, Okayama, Japan
- Monash University, Melbourne, Australia
- Morgagni-Pierantoni Hospital, Forli, Italy
- MTT Agrifood Research Finland, Jokioinen, Finland
- Nagoya City University, Nagoya, Japan
- National Autonomous University of Mexico, Mexico City, Mexico
- National Cancer Institute of Canada, Kingston, Canada
- National Institute for Health and Care Excellence (NICE), London, UK
- National Institute of Chemistry, Ljubliana, Slovenia
- National Institute of Medical Herbalists, Exeter, UK
- National Institute of Mental Health and Neurosciences, Bangalore, India
- National University of Ireland, Galway, Ireland
- New Zealand Institute for Plant & Food Research, Auckland, New Zealand
- Northumbria University, Newcastle upon Tyne, UK
- Norwegian Institute of Public Health, Bergen, Norway
- Osaka City University, Osaka, Japan
- Plant & Food Research, Auckland, New Zealand
- Peking University, Peking, China
- Peninsula College of Medicine and Dentistry, Plymouth, UK
- Plymouth University, Plymouth, UK
- Qingdao University, Qingdao, China
- Queen's Hospital, Burton-on-Trend, UK
- Queensland University of Technology, Brisbane, Australia
- Rakuno Gakuen University, Ebetsu, Japan
- RMIT University, Melbourne, Australia
- Rowett Research Institute, Aberdeen, UK
- Royal Adelaide Hospital, Adelaide, Australia
- Royal Australian College of General Practitioners, Melbourne, Australia
- Royal Hospital for Women, Sydney, Australia
- Ruhr University, Bochum, Germany
- RWTH Aachen, Aachen, Germany
- Sahlgrenska University Hospital, Gothenburg, Sweden
- Science University Malaysia, Minden, Malaysia
- Selcuk University, Konya, Turkey

- Shahid Behesti University of Medical Sciences, Tehran, Iran
- Shanghai Institute of Pharmaceutical Industry, Shanghai, China
- Sheba Medical Center, Ramat Gan, Israel
- Silbersee Paracelsus Hospital, Hanover, Germany
- Skane University Hospital, Malmo, Sweden
- St. Gerardo Hospital, Milan, Italy
- St. George's Hospital Medical School, London, UK
- St. Joseph's Hospital, Hamilton, Canada
- St. Michael's Hospital, Toronto, Canada
- St. Thomas Hospital, London, UK
- Southampton General Hospital, Southampton, UK
- South Australian Research Institute, Adelaide, Australia
- Swansea University, Swansea, UK
- Swedish Research Council, Stockholm, Sweden
- Swinburne University of Technology, Melbourne, Australia
- Swollownest Court Hospital, Sheffield, UK
- Technical University of Darmstadt, Darmstadt, Germany
- Teheran University of Medical Sciences, Teheran, Iran
- Tel-Aviv University, Tel-Aviv, Israel
- Telethon Kids Institute, Perth, Australia
- The Silbersee Paracelsus Hospital, Hannover, Germany
- Thomas Hospital, London, UK
- Tokyo College of Pharmacy, Tokyo, Japan
- Technical University of Darmstadt, Germany
- Toyama Medical and Pharmaceutical University, Toyama, Japan
- Trent University, Peterborough, Canada
- Universidad Camilo Jose Cela, Madrid, Spain
- Universidad de Navarra, Navarra, Spain
- Universidade do Vale do Itajai, Itajai, Brazil
- Universidad Federal da Paraiba, Brazil
- Universite de Montreal, Montreal, Canada
- University College, Cork, Ireland
- University College, London, UK
- University Hospital Jena, Jena, Germany
- University Hospital of Leicester, Leicester, UK
- University of Adelaide, Adelaide, Australia
- University of Athens, Athens, Greece
- University of Basel, Basel, Switzerland
- University of Bern, Bern, Switzerland
- University of Bologna, Bologna, Italy
- University of Bonn, Germany
- University of Bristol, Bristol, UK

- University of British Columbia, Vancouver, Canada
- University of Cambridge, UK
- University of Copenhagen, Denmark
- University of Cordoba, Cordoba, Spain
- University of East Anglia, Norwich, UK
- University of Eastern Finland, Joensuu, Finland
- University of Edinburgh, Edinburgh, UK
- University of Exeter, Exeter, UK
- University of Giessen, Giessen, Germany
- University of Glasgow, Glasgow, UK
- University of Gothenburg, Gothenburg, Sweden
- University of Granada, Granada, Spain
- University of Hong Kong, China
- University of Hull, UK
- University of Las Palmas de Gran Canaria, Las Palmas de Gran Canaria, Spain
- University of Leicester, Leicester, UK
- University of Liverpool, Liverpool, UK
- University of London, London, UK
- University of Lund, Sweden
- University of Maastricht, Maastricht, Netherlands
- University of Madrid, Spain
- University of Malaga, Malaga, Spain
- University of Manchester, Manchester, UK
- University of Medical Sciences, Tehran, Iran
- University of Milan, Milan, Italy
- University of Navarra, Pamplona, Spain
- University of Newcastle, Callaghan, Australia
- University of New South Wales, Sydney, Australia
- University of Otago, Dunedin, New Zealand
- University of Oxford, Oxford, UK
- University of Pavia, Pavia, Italy
- University of Pompeu Fabra, Barcelona, Spain
- University of Portsmouth, Portsmouth, UK
- University of Quality and Efficiency in Health Care, Cologne, Germany
- University of Queensland, Brisbane, Australia
- University of Regensburg, Germany
- University of Sao Paulo, Sao Paulo, Brazil
- University of Sheffield, Sheffield, UK
- University of Shizuoka, Shizuoka, Japan
- University of Singapore, Singapore
- University of Southern Queensland, Darling Heights, Australia

- University of Southampton, Southampton, UK
- University of Surrey, Guildford, UK
- University of Sydney, Sydney, Australia
- University of Tokyo, Tokyo, Japan
- University of Toronto, Toronto, Canada
- University of Tsukuba, Tsukuba, Japan
- University of Ulster, Coleraine, UK
- University of Vienna, Austria
- University of Warwick, Coventry, UK
- University of Western Ontario, London, Canada
- University of Western Sydney, Parramatto, Australia
- University of Wollongong, Wollongong, Australia
- Wageningen University, Wageningen, Netherlands
- Wakayama Medical University, Wakayama, Japan
- Weifang Medical University, Shandong, China
- Weizmann Institute, Rehovot, Israel
- Western General Hospital, Edinburgh, UK
- Women's College Hospital, Toronto
- World Cancer Research Fund, London, UK
- World Health Organization (WHO)
- Yeshiva University, New York City, NY
- Zhejiang University, Hangzhou, China

ABOUT THE AUTHOR

Dr. Mark Fritz, NMD, PhD is licensed in Naturopathy (North Carolina, USA) and President and Founder of New Medical Frontiers, Inc. He has a career as an internationally renowned researcher in the field of holistic ecology and natural medicine. He is also a qualified expert on Natural Medicine in Europe (European Economic Chamber of Trade, Commerce, and Industry).

Based on holistic ecology, it is his mission to focus on the human being as part of the natural environment and the laws of nature men dependent on. He is specializing on information and education in Natural Cancer Support, Chronic Illness, Personalized Health Planning, and Second Medical Opinion - with special reference to renowned U.S. and international medical schools and research institutions.

His Academic Career includes:
Researcher, Max Planck Institute, Munich, Germany; Research Scientist with the United Nations in Paris; Visiting Professor. Oklahoma State University; Adj. Associate Professor & Associate Director of Natural Resources, University of Georgia; Trainee in the Mexican Rainforest.

His Board Certifications are:
American Alternative Medical Association
American Association of Drugless Practitioners
American College of Wellness

>>><<<

If you have any questions, please feel free to contact him personally:

Dr.Mark.Fritz@newmedicalfrontiers.com

>>><<<

New Medical Frontiers, Inc. was founded in January 1999. The focus is on documentation, information and education in the field of Natural Medicine. Today this company has a huge database documenting latest and up-to-date scientific research carried out at renowned U.S. and international medical schools and research institutions.

www.ingramcontent.com/pod-product-compliance
Lightning Source LLC
Chambersburg PA
CBHW072253270326
41930CB00010B/2365